MW01280010

Raw Food
&
Health

By

DR. ST. LOUIS A. ESTES

The Cripple Who Rebuilt Himself

Internationally Known Educator, Author and Publisher

Originator of the Estesian Philosophy of LONGEVITY
Through His Discovery of BRAIN BREATHING
and Dynamic Breath Controls for Disease
Prevention and Life Extension

Father and Founder of the International Back to Nature Raw
Food Movement

International Authority on Old Age and Raw Foods

Raw Food
&
Health

Copyright by DR. ST. LOUIS A. ESTES

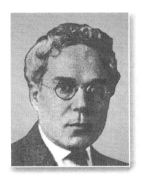

DR. ST. LOUIS A. ESTES

**The man whose marvelous discoveries and teachings
have been revolutionizing the standards of living
throughout the world for the past sixteen years,
and which are helping Millions of People to turn OLD ACE
into youth and Disease into Health.**

Is President of

American Raw Food and Health Association.
International Back to Nature Association.
Estes International Back to Nature Raw Food
and Health Association.
International President of Estes Raw Food and
Health Clubs.
Publisher of Back to Nature Magazine and Raw Food and Health,
published by Estes International Back to Nature Raw Food
and Health Association, an international scientific organization
for Public Education.
Teaching how to live 150 years by Back to Nature Methods.

Dedication

In loving memory of my mother and sister, whose untimely death was the incentive which spurred me on to attain a greater knowledge of Life and Health, that I might help others to be spared the grief which I suffered through the early loss of my dear ones, this book is dedicated.

St. Louis A. Estes

CONTENTS

Author's Preface

The author's object in writing this book is to give to the laity and those of the profession who are sufficiently interested, the benefit of his own experience in overcoming disease by natural methods of living.

The teachings herein are the outgrowth of experiments and research worked out on myself several years ago after I had been given up to die from diseases of varied character and severity which involved my entire body.

I was born and raised in the South, where the dining table groaned under the weight of rich, highly-seasoned and fried foods which were served three times a day, with hearty refreshment between these meals a regular occurrence.

I have made a practical application of my teachings on myself, family and patients, and I feel, therefore, that I am qualified to expound the merits of natural methods of living for the benefit of those whose fruitless quest for health has brought them only disappointment and despair.

It is my great hope that doctors, dentists and the laity in general will find information within these pages which will be of great practical use to them in their daily life.

I do not protest against vegetarianism or fruitarianism or any other system of living, for the purpose of argument or from motives of unworthy prejudice and biased conviction. I only point out the deficiencies of all modes of living when those modes do not succeed in achieving their purpose and where they do not build strong and perfect Health.

The Divine mind has in Its infinite wisdom provided the human family with foods which are perfect in their composition and of sufficient variety and character to meet all the needs of the human body. Man, in his egotism, attempts to improve upon the product of the Creator. The result is disease and death.

Man in his original state knew nothing of fires, cook stoves, cooked foods, calories and heat units. His strength and prowess then were greater than they have been since. Long use of cooked, highly-seasoned foods have deprived man of his natural instincts in the selection of foods. The taste buds of the tongue have become atrophied and the appetites perverted.

The present-day cooked foods, demineral-ized, refined and devitalized, breed only pestilence and early death.

When living on Raw Foods it is not necessary to know the calories, heat units and chemical composition of foods, for the raw food diet with nuts, fruits and milk equalizes and balances itself. It is only because the foods are cooked that their power is destroyed, and it is necessary to calculate the units of heat and energy which they contain in order to combine them so as to afford the strength necessary to the body.

It is an erroneous idea that certain fruits, berries and vegetables are poisonous to some individuals. These foods are not poisonous in themselves. It is the individual's system which is poisoned, and the fruit, berry or vegetable which distresses him simply possesses the mineral element which is necessary to eliminate that poison. Hence, we find rashes, boils, eruptions, blotches and other disturbances which are only manifested when certain foods are eaten. It is far wiser to continue the use of these foods for a time and eliminate the poisons of the body than to take drugs which drive them into the system.

All diseases are originally produced in bodies which are starved—starved for food, starved for air, starved for sunshine, sleep, water, exercise and oxygen.

If mothers would confine themselves to the pure and nutritious foods, with few combinations, not exceeding two or three at a meal, we could soon produce a super race.

It is the great variety and injudicious combinations of food which cause trouble. The chemical reaction necessary to take care of the different foods produces acid which breaks down the body and causes disease.

On a diet of clean, wholesome foods, eaten in their natural live state, the system is kept free from fermentation and clogging impurities, which poison and deplete. The sensibilities become keener and more delicate, the temperament more pliable and docile, the mind more alert and receptive to new ideas, and the character, molded by these influences, becomes more noble and the soul more exalted.

We are created to render service to humanity, and this service can only be rendered in the highest degree when we have developed the Spiritual, Mental and Physical. Spiritual and Mental advancement are achieved only in proportion to the physical development. We can develop perfect physical bodies and robust health through right living.

Let us gaze into the mirror of life, view ourselves as we should be and as we are, and with the roadway cleared before us, let us, with new courage and determination, set out to reach the great goal Health, which insures Happiness and Harmony to all who possess it.

The Author

Dr. Estes Slogans:
"To Be a Deep Thinker You Must Be a Deep Breather"
"As Man Breatheth, So Will He Be"
"You Are As Old As Your Blood"
"Your Health Is Your Wealth"
"As a Man Eateth, So Is He"
"Talk Less, Think More"
"How to Live 150 Years"

RAW FOOD AND HEALTH

Eat and absorb LIFE as Nature has provided it, that you may have long life, youth and happiness.

This book is compiled to assist and guide those who are endeavoring to regain or retain their health through the use of natural foods. By Natural Foods I mean foods which are eaten in their natural state—uncooked or raw. Some individuals protest against the term Raw Food as differentiated from Uncooked Food, stating that Raw Food is unfit to eat and, therefore, unhealthful, as for instance a green apple is raw whereas a ripe apple is not "Raw" but merely "Unfired." However, I assume that my readers and patients have, at least, ordinary intelligence and will not be prone to misconstrue my meaning when I allude to Raw Food. For the sake of simplicity, I prefer the term "Raw." To me it suggests fresh, green salads, crisp vegetables, and luscious fruits, none of which have been subjected to the devastating heat of the flame and the consequent devitalizing changes which destroy its freshness and render it so much waste when taken into the human system.

Many people are anxious to live upon raw food but are at a loss to know the relative merits of each article of

unfired food and what combinations to employ. While I
have studiously avoided the field of food chemistry and
have kept the book free from technicalities, I have
attempted to outline the principles of a raw food diet so
that those who have suffered from previous dietetic errors
may profit by my own personal research and experience.
The subject is a vast one and it would be impossible to
completely cover it in a book of this size. However, I have
set down enough concise facts, suggestions, and menus to
be of great assistance to the average reader.

Four essential factors for Health are Oxygenation,
Food, Assimilation and Elimination. Food is what one
authority has defined as anything that can be chewed and
swallowed. Few people take their food seriously. They eat
at 8, 12, 6, whether they are hungry or not creatures of
habit, they gravitate toward home or a restaurant at a given
hour and proceed to overload a stomach which has been
tired from infancy and long ago laid down on a job that
was far too strenuous. If the human race should succeed in
forever casting out the erroneous conviction that it is not
sufficiently or properly nourished at a meal until it has
distended its stomach to the point of bursting, then we
might begin to have intelligent material, fit to mould into
sound, healthy beings. Foods are divided into three classes,
Builders, Heat Generators, Intestinal Cleansers and
Eliminators. I. The building foods must of necessity carry
protein since the proteins create energy and power and
restore and nourish the tissues. Foremost in this class are
eggs, milk, nuts and the whole grains. II. The heat
generating foods carry sugar, oils and starch. By sugar, I do
not mean the highly refined sugar which we use in candy,
cakes and pastries but the organic sugars contained in
fruits, such as grapes, bananas, figs and dates. The
chemical reaction of this organic sugar is vastly different
from the acid-generating, commercial sugar eaten in
cooked sweets, candy and ice cream. Oils we obtain from

nuts, butter and cream, ripe olives and olive oil. A certain quantity of starch is essential but the greatest trouble with the average person's diet is that he eats too much starch. It is a common sight to see people in restaurants eating meat, potatoes, baked beans and spaghetti and white bread, pie or a tart for dessert, with no salad, fruit or green vegetable to offset the effects of this starchy heavy meal. This is not an exaggeration either. I have personally observed meals of this and similar kinds placed before individuals, one person actually eating all of the above named articles. The action of raw starch presents a radical contrast to that of the cooked starches. Raw potatoes, corn and peas eaten sparingly provide the system with the necessary starch but do not lay in the stomach in a heavy indigestible mass which causes fermentation and gas. III. The intestinal cleansers and eliminators are the watery vegetables, the green leafy vegetables and the juicy, acid fruits, all rich in organic salts, lettuce, spinach, cabbage, celery, water-cress, etc. No meal should be eaten (unless it is a fruit or nut meal entirely) without a salad or one of the green vegetables. The purifying and stimulating effects of these greens and vegetables are invaluable and if real health is desired, they must form an important part in the general diet.

Water—Although the layman does not consider it so and few physicians regard its merits in a serious light, water is a food in itself. If we drank more water and flushed the system thoroughly, we should have fewer operations for gall stones, kidney and bladder stones, and adhesions. Seventy-five per cent of the human body is water. Does this not prove conclusively that we need a constant supply of water to purify the bloodstream, stimulate the tissues and replenish the water which is constantly carrying off the poisons? Since water is one-half oxygen and we cannot live unless we breathe oxygen, is it not reasonable to believe that the inner organs of our bodies, the tissues and nerves and delicate membranes, require oxygen to sustain them? No water, in fact no liquid of any kind, should be taken with a cooked meal, as it retards the action of the salivary ducts, drenches the food and reduces its temperature, making it necessary for the stomach to heat the food to the required bodily temperature before the digestive processes begin. Detailed instructions in the correct use of water, externally and internally, will be found further on in this book.

Many people smile indulgently when I say I live on Raw Food. They think I am a fanatic or a faddist. The fact which has struck me so forcibly in incidents of this character is that the people who smile in their superior way and are not interested or even curious enough to ask questions, are the very individuals whose bodies are over-fed and diseased or undernourished and dried-up. They are the people who most need enlightenment on food and instruction in body rebuilding. But since one only gains the reputation of being a bore when he attempts to enlighten those who do not desire enlightenment, I can only go my way and reserve my energy for those who continually seek knowledge and assistance as they progress in search of Health.

In changing one's diet, particularly when attempting to use Raw Food to the exclusion of all else, I would warn against a too abrupt change from cooked food to raw food. I have had experiences which make it necessary for me to admonish people to employ some common sense. One case in particular, a seemingly intelligent woman of mature years, heard one of my lectures on Raw Food. As I learned later, she went home wedded to the idea.

The following morning she ground up several pounds of cabbage, onions, carrots and mostly everything that was available, I think. She ate a huge bowl of this vegetable mash for breakfast, another bowl for lunch, and a third for dinner. That night she became so distended with gas and was seized with such violent cramps that it was necessary to summon a doctor.

Of course, the lady's intentions were commendable as was her determination, but she failed sadly in her judgment. In her zeal to do the correct thing she committed the error of eating a poor combination and too large a quantity, with the result that she was so disgusted with the results it was difficult to convince her after all that a Raw Food Diet could possibly have any advantages.

Obviously, no one could relish eating a mass of the same crushed vegetables three times a day. It is like feeding swill to a pig. It is far better to select and eat one or two articles of food, have them fresh, crisp and appetizing and rich in their distinctive values than to crush and combine them with other vegetables and expose them to the air, thereby losing some of their nutritive properties and reducing them all to a homogeneous mass which appeals to neither the eye nor palate. The instant that a vegetable or fruit is crushed and exposed to the air, just that instant does a cellular change take place and some of the food value is consequently lost, the amount depending upon the length of time the article stands before consumption.

Sudden changes of diet may have serious results; the age, physical condition, susceptibility to food reactions, and the general nerve conditions must all be considered. It is safest to change the diet gradually. If you have been eating principally meat and potatoes, eliminate the meat and substitute a vegetable and a salad, or if you cannot abstain totally from meat cut it down to two or three times a week until you gradually break away from it. Meanwhile cultivate and encourage a taste for the various vegetables, particularly those which are ordinarily eaten uncooked. Many people are not naturally fond of salads, lettuce, tomatoes, etc., and for these people the Raw Diet represents a great problem. Since they are not fond of the foods which everyone eats raw, how can they educate themselves to a completely raw diet?   Only by a concentrated idea that they are benefiting themselves in every way, that they are breaking away from habits established centuries ago and practiced by millions of people who go to early graves as a result of the foods they eat, only by a determined effort to give themselves a fair chance, can they succeed in conquering an unwholesome appetite and winning a victory over palate and nose.

If meat has already been eliminated then the progress is more rapid, for every vegetarian knows how much better he has felt since he ceased to eat flesh and he is therefore more receptive to advanced ideas on food than is the individual who clings to his meat as a surly dog to a bone. It is, with few exceptions, difficult to convince people that they may abstain from meat and contrive to live more than a few days. In fact most people firmly believe if they miss a meal they are one step nearer the grave, whereas in most cases each meal they eat shortens their lives by so many days or weeks. When they learn that meat is dead material, an animal corpse, carrying all the poisons which infested the living animal at the time it was killed, and that it is only so much fibrous waste matter which calls forth all the reserve strength of the system for expulsion; when they learn that the reason they feel stronger after eating meat is because the body is exerting every effort to rid itself of the poison and is summoning every atom of energy to aid in the process, thus producing a superficial stimulation which makes the individual feel stronger for a time but later leaves him with a hollow, weak feeling; then they find they cannot only live without meat but they can live without cooked food, then the path to Good Health is cleared of the underbrush and the way is comparatively smooth. Research shows that the *meat-eating Indians lived only about sixty years* while the *nut* and *maize-eating Indians* reached the mature age of from 126 *to* 180 *years*. Statistics prove that Raw Food induces longevity.

We owe it not only to ourselves but to the world to build up fine, healthy bodies and keen active minds, and prolong our lives to the utmost in order to render the *greatest service we can to humanity.* Scientists tell us now that when we leave this planet and pass into the next world we take up work there according to the stage of development we have achieved here. If this be true, it should be an added incentive to spur us on to the highest pinnacles of *mental, physical* and *spiritual perfection.*

Let me impress my readers with this fact: If you once come to a full realization of the merits of raw food, if you can visualize your alimentary tract as a clean, wholesome part of your anatomy instead of a dark and gloomy recess packed with putrified, *gaseous masses of undigested food*, if you can teach your sense of taste and smell that it is only the salt and pepper in the meat and other cooked food which makes it palatable at all and that if you had to eat these same foods without seasoning of any kind, you would promptly reject them (if you don't believe it—try it), then you are striding along the path of victory and you have conquered your tongue and your nose.

When you learn to appreciate the flavor of crisp vegetables and salads and understand that every mouthful you eat is creating new energy and power, and is purifying your entire system until you are as clean internally as you should be externally, then you will be unable to slip back, even occasionally, to your old diet of cooked foods without a twinge of conscience because you will know that you are injuring yourself. You will have a mental picture of what is taking place in your clean stomach and colon when you crowd them with rare steak, fried potatoes, pie and coffee, and your conscience will squirm in a most annoying way.

You will have lost your capacity to enjoy a conventional meal, that is, of course, if *Health* means anything to you, and this book is only written for the benefit of those who seek Health. When I am able to penetrate your *gustatory calm* and disturb your dietetic equilibrium to a point where a mental question mark punctuates every meal, then

I shall have you treading the primrose path to Health and Happiness.

It is a fallacy to suppose that the only requisite for Health is a correct diet. Many people studiously seek a corrective diet, and having found it, or feeling convinced they have found it, they proceed to eat that particular food, sit back and calmly await complete rejuvenation. When their lost youth fails to materialize they become disheartened and cynical and turn again to their old habits of eating. Food is not the only essential to life—true, we must eat but we must also *breathe* and exercise. While the proper food will nourish and build the body, it must have oxygen to strengthen and revivify, and exercise to stimulate.

MAL-NUTRITION—MAN'S COMMON ENEMY

Malnutrition is a malady more prevalent, perhaps, than any other disease with the possible exception of constipation. We find malnutrition in the young and old, thin and fat. It is due to either one or two things or both—an incorrect diet or imperfect assimilation of the food. Many people are scrupulously careful with regard to their diet, but do not realize the importance of thorough mastication, without which there can be no perfect assimilation.

Mal-nutrition, as most people understand it, is a disease which is indicated in cases of extreme anemia, general weakness and debility. This disease is by no means restricted to frail, delicate people, but those of apparently good health are often unconscious victims of it.

Symptoms of mal-nutrition. There are two distinctive types which illustrate the effects of malnutrition. The best-known type is the thin, emaciated individual with dried, leathery skin, soft, flabby muscles and a lean, gaunt look. These people usually have a great deal of nerve energy, that is to say, they appear to have. In reality, their nervous systems are badly depleted, but they force every atom of energy to the surface and keep themselves going on the effects of what reserve they have.

They are always at high tension, are nervous, irritable, easily agitated and very highly sensitive to pain. The eyes are pale and watery, showing the continual draining of the lachrymal gland, and the hair is dry and scant. This type is inordinately fond of either sweets or sour foods, such as pickles and relishes of all kinds—the two extremes. They bolt their food with little or no mastication or else they spend much time over it but fail even then to chew it enough to render it assimilable.

I have found by close observation in my years of practice that these cases invariably have, among other diseases, advanced pyorrhea. The impoverished bloodstream is unable to convey sufficient nourishment to the jaws and teeth, and the result is the gradual breaking down and ultimate destruction of gums, teeth and jawbone.

They also develop such diseases as intestinal *cancer, asthma, hay fever, anemia* and various ailments too numerous to mention. Let it be said, also, that this type is especially fond of salt.

Treatment. To correct this depleted physical condition the patients should be put on a rich, nourishing diet of which milk and cream will form a very important part. The addition of plenty of green vegetables and fruits will supply the deficiency of mineral salts, and the copious use of water internally will oxygenate and expand the dried tissues. Fresh air and sunlight, with as much sleep as it is possible to get, at least ten hours each night, will go far towards effecting a rapid recovery and the establishment of sound, vigorous health.

Other symptoms: The second type of malnutrition is the opposite extreme. Fat and flabby with a soft, pudgy appearance, they are sometimes sallow and pale, sometimes fair and flushed. They present a bloated appearance which deceives themselves and many others into thinking they are in a state of perfect health. The practiced eye of the physician, however, is able to discern the difference between the unwholesome, flabby flesh of disease and the firm, solid flesh of health. These types are fond of rich, highly-seasoned foods, pastries and sweets and all foods rich in protein and starches. They are eating constantly and lead lazy, inactive lives. By inactive lives I mean they move slowly, exert themselves as little as possible and never engage in strenuous exercise. The foods which they eat all go to build the destructive cells which form the degenerated fat tissue that constitutes their weight. Due to the individual's inactivity, the rich foods are not assimilated, but lie in the stomach and intestines, where they putrefy and decompose. The destructive fat cells are able to absorb enough nourishment from this unassimilated food to keep on increasing and growing, but the healthy cells of the nerve and muscle tissues are unable to derive sufficient nourishment to build the strength and energy which are necessary to vitally healthy bodies. The rapidly multiplying fat cells sap the reserve energy from the other parts of the body and cause the individual to be phlegmatic, lethargic and mentally sluggish. Persons of this class are usually self-satisfied, predisposed to gossip and perverted ideas resulting from a general physical depression due to the absorption of toxic poisons in the body. They have little endurance but are long-lived, because their consistent inactivity makes no demand on what little reserve energy they store up. They are necessarily people of limited accomplishments and frequently of a warped mentality, since a brain fed by a poisonous bloodstream has small opportunity for full development.

Cooked food vs. malnutrition: The treatment in all cases of malnutrition is manifestly a diet carrying 100% nutrition accompanied by exercise, fresh air and a cheerful mental attitude. Raw foods are the only foods which carry 100% nutrition with the full quota of vitamins. This cannot be truthfully stated of foods which have been cooked. Alfred McCann, the pure food expert, has stated that from the average meal only 6% nutrition is derived—the remaining percentage is waste, which the body eliminates or retains, according to its condition. If this excess waste is eliminated, the body is, of course, in a cleaner condition and not so subject to auto-intoxication, which adds to the miseries of malnutrition, as the body which retains much of the waste and re-absorbs the poisons therefrom. When we consider that the majority of people are deprived of just 94% of the nourishment they should have, it is no wonder that we see emaciated weaklings all around us who drag on from day to day, stuffing themselves with food but never increasing in power and efficiency.

Raw food to reduce: The phlegmatic person will find raw foods of the greatest value in breaking down unhealthy fat tissue and replacing it with firm flesh, the amount of which may be easily regulated. Raw, green vegetables and juicy-fruits are the certain enemies of flabby, diseased flesh, and the unsightly rolls of fat on the shoulders, abdomen and hips, as well as the girth of the waist, will be rapidly reduced on a diet of raw foods. Effective reducing is quickly accomplished with raw foods without sustaining the sunken-faced, hollow-eyed look which usually characterizes the man or woman who attempts to reduce by starving himself on a meager diet of cooked foods which, when eaten plentifully, carry the minimum amount of nutrition. When that minimum is cut, slow starvation sets in.

Raw food a corrective: Raw foods are the specific cure for malnutrition. Where the forces of the body are lowered through lack of proper nourishment, energizing foods which will restore the strength and vitality are needed. Plenty of water taken before and between meals to flush the system, healthful exercise, sleep, and as much fresh air as possible will aid materially in overcoming the most stubborn cases of malnutrition.

Malnutrition, as its name implies, is simply poor nutrition of the body—undernourishment, a form of slow starvation. Animals and plants cannot resist the proper nourishment if administered under favorable conditions; neither can the nerves and tissues of the body resist the proper kinds of foods if they are fed on them. The response is gratifying, and, once gained, improvement is astonishingly rapid.

COLDS ARE TO BE FEARED

The cure of the most prolific thief of the universe, the old fashioned, every day cold, is so simple that it seems unreasonable that the human race continues to go along blissfully ignorant, satisfied to believe that a cold must run its course and that it must suffer all sorts of misery and discomfort when the remedy is always close at hand.

This monstrous disease stalks about in the guise of an innocent but disagreeable affliction, while in reality it is directly and indirectly responsible for the filling of more graveyards than all the other diseases combined.

How often you hear the remark, "Oh, I'm all right but I have a cold." The individual smiles regretfully and passes on to another subject unless he is the kind who enjoys discussing the slightest ailment at great length, as most people do. Many people seem to take great pride in clinging to a cold for weeks and sometimes months.

A cold should be given immediate attention at the very beginning, with the first sneeze if possible. A congested cold in the head leads to filthy, odious conditions in the nasal passages and the sinuses, and the resultant poisons back up through the entire body. The filth from a cold accumulates inside the body, the same as the dirt on your face and hands. You certainly wash your face if it gets dirty, then why not take the time to cleanse the inside of your body when the process is so simple?

Instead of holding up a congested, poisoned body for the world's observation as though it were a jewel, it would be far more advantageous to eliminate all disease and build the body and health to a high point. It is most disgusting to observe the pride which some people seem to take in parading their ailments. If they would devote the time, spent in minute discussion of their afflictions, to studying their bodies and the conditions which give rise to their diseases, they would be greatly improved and then when they chose to parade themselves before the world and call attention to themselves, their clean, wholesome, healthy bodies would be objects of admiration. They could then shout as loud as they cared to, so the world would learn the secrets which they had found out. This procedure would *help* humanity.

Colds are produced by the *waste* of cooked food-poisons which are not being carried off. These poisons accumulate rapidly when the refuse of the system is retained and the body becomes surcharged with the noxious gases and poisonous vapors which generate in the clogged intestines and infiltrate the bloodstream and all the nerves and tissues. Did you ever consult a physician about a cold that he didn't inquire about the condition of your bowels?

This stagnant condition of the bowels, having its effect on the bloodstream, lowers the circulation and undermines the resistance. If the body is subjected to the slightest change of temperature or exposed to a current of chill air for a few moments, the circulation, already lowered, is practically checked altogether. The congestion which takes place is reflected over the entire body and before long you are sneezing and coughing, the air passages of the head are restricted and closed up; the nerves of the eyes are weakened, the ears ring and general misery envelopes the sufferer.

I was a continual sufferer with colds for years. At the be-ginning of every fall my head began to congest. I sneezed, coughed and was generally miserable. This condition ex-isted through the winter and lasted until spring.

I was forced to resort to all kinds of douches, snuff, washes, drugs and any and all palliatives or reputed cures which would relieve me in any degree.

My doctor friends, and I had a number of them, were kept busy. I had one friend in particular, God bless him, who took me in hand like a fond mother at the beginning of the season, and with the patience of a saint he strove to find a remedy to help me. He nearly wore out his eyes hunting up remedies to alleviate the conditions in my worn-out, diseased carcass. He is one of the few who survived and he ranks among the foremost practitioners and diagnosticians of today. The others succumbed to disease and went the way of all flesh. Perhaps his endurance was augmented when I lifted the weight of my burden from his shoulders and assumed my part in trying to overcome my chronic ailments by endeavoring to build my general health and improve my physical development.

I found the moment I learned to draw air, oxygen (the breath of life), into the head, I burnt up the catarrhal conditions in the head. I had heard of the necessity for deep breathing, but with the lethargy which characterizes most people, I paid no attention to it and made no effort to apply the principles to myself until I became so desperate that I had to decide whether I was to die or go on living in abject misery. I decided to do neither: I studied out the situation and determined to eliminate the poisonous conditions which made me a victim of every breath of air that touched me.

I began to practice deep breathing, but while I found the systems of breathing generally beneficial, I felt that they were limited in their possibilities. Accordingly, I began a long, laborious study of the respiratory organs and the action of the oxygen upon the various parts of the body.

After years of study *I succeeded in working out a system of breathing* which involved the bowels, abdomen, thoracic cavity, intercostal muscles and nerves, face, head and frontal sinus, ethmoid and sphenoid bones, nasal cavity and antrum and brain. The perfect *oxygenation* of each of these parts was effected, and the uniting of the various breaths formed the sum total, *the complete and perfect breath.*

Thus, every part of the body is oxygenated from the top of the brain to the rectum.

By drawing the air deeply into the body, the *oxygen* can be forced through the tissues, reaching the brain cells, the head cavities, distending the tiny veins and muscles of the *shoulders, neck, back, wrists, arms, hands* and even the *limbs, ankles* and *feet,* This constitutes *complete breathing*.

This system is the only one known today which embraces *all* of the *organs* in one *breath*. It is being extensively used in correcting all organic disorders, constipation and diseases of the head. If systematically practiced, it becomes a uniform, automatic procedure and eventually impregnates the subconscious mind and becomes a part of the bodily functioning. It stimulates the circulation and purifies the blood.

Becoming encouraged with the results of my early experience in breathing, I began to study the action of foods and found that the less food I ate when I had a cold the better I felt and the sooner I improved.   Orange juice and fresh water comprised my diet when an acute condition developed. I alternated them and drank a glass of each from one-half to an hour apart By drawing about five deep breaths of air into the head every two hours, I succeeded in loosening the congestion. I made it a point to be out of doors in the fresh air and sunshine as much as possible *so* that all the air I breathed was pure and fresh. Sitting and sleeping in a close, warm room are bad enough at any time, but are particularly injurious when any congestion of the head is present.

As my condition steadily improved, the colds came on less and less frequently. I took up the matter of foods, solid foods, seriously, and by close observation and personal experiment, I came to know the evils of cooked, demineralized foods, which bloat and corrupt the body and destroy health and life.

Since I have learned *how to live*, I am free from colds, fatigue and other diseases to which the human body is subject.

So-called simple coughs and colds often develop into fatal diseases.

Tuberculosis, influenza, chronic bronchitis, pleurisy, pneumonia, grippe, lumbago, neuralgia, sinus troubles, chronic eye, ear, nose and throat diseases, catarrh, laryngitis, uteroovarian troubles, sciatica, rheumatism and other serious maladies are often brought on by the congestion and stagnation due to a neglected cold.

A long-standing cough is a source of irritation to the entire system. The nerves become worn and fatigued; the individual loses ambition and interest, is sluggish, stupid and morose. The vitality is sapped by the continual drain on the nerves, and the body is rendered susceptible to almost any disease.

Don't neglect a cold: Don't get it in the first place if you can help it. Keep your body clean internally and externally. Build your health, purify your bloodstream with *oxygen and natural live foods.*

If you contract a cold before you have learned how to live properly, don't let it run on indefinitely.

Get as much fresh air as possible.

Exercise before an open window and inhale deeply. Drive the *oxygen* up into the head, hold it a few seconds and force it out with an explosive action.

Sleep with the windows open.

Don't bundle up unnecessarily. Have the clothing warm but loose, so the skin can eliminate thoroughly.

Bathe frequently and follow the bath with a quick chilling by splashing cold water over the body with a spray or wet cloth. This closes the pores, prevents the contraction of more cold and stimulates the circulation.

Keep the bowels open with a good mineral oil. Constipation aggravates cold conditions and the retention of the poisons superinduces serious complications.

Flush the kidneys with plenty of water. Remember, the kidneys and bowels, lungs and skin are all eliminators. See that they all function actively.

Do not crowd or overload the stomach.

Let fruit juices comprise the diet until the cold is greatly mitigated. Drink the juices freely and whenever hungry.

COFFEE AND TEA
–DISEASE PRODUCERS–

"Animals eat only what is good and wholesome.
Horses and dogs shun what is injurious."

The American people depend more and more upon coffee as a part of their diet. It is the regulation beverage, and without it no breakfast, luncheon or dinner is complete. Afternoon tea, a custom exclusively English, but which we frankly ape, is satisfying to the ladies, who find it soothing after a harrowing day of bargain hunting, or use it as an excuse for the exchange of social amenities.

But catch any he-man drinking tea with his meals, unless his physician has bluffed him into it. No, indeed, he must have strong, black coffee, at least one or two cups, and often three or four.

Many people who would prefer to drink coffee three times a day compromise with themselves by taking tea at one meal, for somewhere in a remote corner of their brain they are inclined to credit some of the facts which are circulated regarding coffee. They give themselves a free hand with the tea, and because well-brewed tea is erroneously considered less harmful than coffee, they drink twice the amount of it.

Caffeine and Theine. The active principle of tea and coffee is the same, but in *coffee* it is called caffeine, while in tea it is called theine. Practically the only difference between the effects of tea and coffee is that it requires larger doses of theine than caffeine to produce the same results. Both are cerebro-spinal stimulants, which stimulate first and paralyze afterward. Caffeine acts directly upon the motor nerves, while theine affects the sensory nerves.

Theine decreases the bodily temperature— caffeine increases it. The caffeine or theine in tea is an alkaloid which if administered in doses of from three to five grains pro-

duces wakefulness. Larger doses cause intense wakefulness, mental unrest and great restlessness and trembling
muscles. Toxic doses paralyze the heart. *The symptoms of
caffeine or theine poison* are: Buzzing in the ears, flashes of
light, congested feeling in the head, feeble pulse, coldness
of surface temperature of body and increased central temperature. Even moderate quantities of tea and coffee will
frequently cause an irregularity in the heartbeat with some
people, particularly those who are not accustomed to
drinking these beverages. *Coffee contains two to three grains
of caffeine* to each cup. The quantity of *theine* contained in
one *cup of tea* is about *four-fifths of a grain, or one-quarter* of a
medicinal dose, which is three and one-fifth grains.   The
amount of theine or caffeine which the average person consumes at a meal may be quickly computed.   When you
consider that this drug is administered medicinally only
when a powerful stimulant is required, it seems amazing
that the tea and coffee addicts can so ruthlessly ply themselves with a drug which even physicians employ with discretion.   Caffeine is used as a part of the treatment in some
forms of heart depression, nervous afflictions, opium nar-
cosis and the insomnia of extreme alcoholism. If taken in
moderate amounts it increases the blood pressure, stimulates the brain and increases the reasoning power and
spurs the imagination.   It is sometimes given credit for aug-
menting the muscular strength, but it is apparent on the
surface that such a condition, if really existing, would only
be the result of extreme artificial stimulation and could not
long endure.   It is true, however, that many students and
workers rely upon the effects of coffee and tea to force
themselves on through an arduous task. The student cram-
ming for an examination burns the midnight oil and drinks
quantities of black coffee. While it may seem absurd to
mention it here, the fact has been called to my attention
that a great many laundresses seem content with a small
amount of food if they have plenty of tea or coffee. They

will wash and iron day after day, standing on their feet nine hours at a stretch, and practically their only sustenance is one of the stimulating beverages mentioned above. These cases may be exceptional, but a number have been cited to me by reliable acquaintances. In each instance the woman was the slight, rather nervous type who worked feverishly and accomplished far more than the stalwart, slow-moving individual who demanded more food. Of course, only a complete collapse faces these hard-working women, who are so poorly informed as to how to care for themselves, but remonstrance provokes only a good-natured smile, and they are on their busy way.

Tea and coffee causes of constipation. Tea due to its astringent properties, is often the cause of chronic constipation. Coffee contains less of the astringent quality, and, due to the presence of aromatic oil, it often tends to stimulate peristalsis. However, a vast amount of colonic and rectal trouble is due to excessive coffee drinking, as after continued use the coffee has a tendency to contract the bowels and dry their natural secretions, so necessary to proper functioning.

Theine is given as an analgesic in the treatment of neuralgia, lumbago and locomotor ataxia. It exercises a prolonged influence over the sensory nerves, paralyzing them and thereby correcting the sensation of pain. This explains why you are so often appreciably helped by a cup of tea when you are suffering from a severe headache. You have simply paralyzed the congested nerves temporarily and gained relief.

The action of tea and coffee on the stomach seems to vary but negligibly. It is after they leave the stomach and are absorbed from the bowel that their injurious effects are to be most readily observed and the variation in action noted. The rapid pulse, nervous tremor and disturbed sleep are less pronounced in the use of tea than in coffee unless, of course, the infusion of tea is extremely strong and large quantities are taken. As a matter of fact, the tea leaf really contains more caffeine or theine than the coffee bean, but because less tea is used in making the beverage, it naturally has a less pronounced effect.

Both tea and coffee act directly upon the kidneys. The diuretic action (effect on the kidneys) of tea is felt almost immediately, and because of this nuisance I have known of one or two cases which were happily forced to abandon the use of tea.

Effects of tannic acid: The tannic acid contained in tea shrinks and warps the nerves and dries the natural oils and secretions of the body. The excessive tea drinker will generally have a dry skin of somewhat leathery texture, which falls into tiny lines and wrinkles very early in life. These tea addicts, like the coffee drunkards, are usually at high tension, being of extremely nervous and irritable temperaments.

Nursing mothers: Expectant and nursing mothers should use neither of these stimulating drinks, since the kidneys before and after childbirth are subject to an unusual strain and should not be further exerted through artificial stimulation. Tea and coffee dilute the milk of the nursing mother, and it is undesirable to have caffeine or theine reach the child through this or any other medium.

Iced tea and coffee: It is a fallacy to suppose that iced tea or coffee have lost any of their exciting properties. They are just as active stimulants as when they are taken piping hot. The stomach at once begins the process of raising their icy temperature to accommodate its own heat, and "then the fun begins."

Effects on digestion: Whether cream or sugar is used in coffee and tea is of little consequence as far as the action of the drinks is concerned. The fat in the cream and the acid of the white sugar only lend additional impetus toward impairing the digestion, causing fermentation, acid and sour stomach. Under no consideration should *children* be permitted coffee or tea. It arrests their growth and development and seriously interferes with their mental activities.

Effects of tea and coffee: The system seems to tolerate excessive coffee drinking in earlier life, particularly if the constitution is reasonably strong. Few, if any, alarming effects are noticed, although many chronic ailments of supposedly minor importance could be traced to the tea and coffee habit. Sensitiveness of the sympathetic nerve is one symptom which had well be corrected, as its neglect leads to serious impingement in the pelvic terminal branches. The correction, of course, would necessitate the diminished use of coffee or a complete abstinence. In early middle age, many reflexes of the sympathetic nerve are due to coffee and tea; the action of the heart is greatly increased, and it is said that the stimulating qualities of coffee have a tendency to excite the sex impulses. On the other hand, the excessive use of coffee is said to be responsible for early *sex impotency*, because it has caused over-stimulation and functioning of the sex organs, to begin with. The over-functioning of any organ for an extended period is always followed by an almost complete cessation of function.

The inveterate coffee drinker generally is distinguished by a pale, sallow complexion or a yellow, saffron-like skin. It would appear in some cases that the tiniest cells of the skin were impregnated with the bilious-hued beverage of the breakfast, lunch and dinner table, so nearly does the complexion resemble that of the famous liquid.

The coffee industry is a thriving one and is constantly growing. Millions of pounds of coffee are imported to the United States alone every year.

Neither coffee nor tea possesses any nutritive value. People depend upon their stimulating properties alone. When we consider how powerfully stimulating they are, it is no wonder that the habitual coffee drinker staggers around in the morning, complains of dizziness, faintness and an "all-gone" feeling if he goes without his coffee. Like any other dope fiend, he naturally misses his dose of dope. He hasn't had his morning shot of caffeine, consequently he isn't up to the mark until he gets it.

Tea and coffee vs. alcohol and tobacco: It is easy enough for the reformers to declaim the evils of alcohol and tobacco, but while I countenance neither, I can well imagine the howl of chagrin if someone in turn proposed that a ban be placed on coffee and tea and appealed for the enforcement of a law against these beverages. The tea and coffee drinkers who admit that they just must have tea and coffee—can't get along without them—do not regard themselves as addicted to a drug. They are moral, self-respecting citizens of temperate habits, yet they must have their daily doses of caffeine and theine or they are not equal to their tasks. They all boast that they could stop drinking tea and coffee if they wanted to, but they never want to. They won't admit the evils of the tea and coffee habit—often they don't know them—but even if these evil effects are pointed out to them, they remain serenely unconcerned in most cases.

It seems to be the thing in popular fiction to chronicle, along with the hero's adventures, his indulgence in coffee. Apropos of a lecture I delivered on coffee, a patient laughingly mentioned a popular novel she had just read, wherein the characters were constantly thwarting the progress of the plot by stopping for a sandwich and coffee or waffles and coffee or lingering over their after-dinner coffee. It was always coffee. This particular patient was very fond of coffee, and she said the book made her so hungry by its constant references to coffee that she had difficulty restraining herself from humoring her appetite.

As England is a tea-drinking country, so is America the land of coffee addicts, and while afternoon coffee, which the Germans and Scandinavians enjoy, apparently has not become a prevalent habit here, the ritual of the coffee cup is an iron-clad rule to be observed at breakfast, luncheon and dinner in the average American household.

Little wonder that we are degenerating into a race of hysterical, dyspeptics, harassed with various ills and ailments, our nerves depleted, irritable and unstrung, when we are steadily feeding our bodies on demineralized foods which slowly kill, and when these bodies are half dead we animate them daily with powerful drugs and artificial stimulants in the guise of harmless table beverages.

In isolated cases, coffee has caused intoxication. The author had a patient a few years ago who said that one cup of coffee had the effect of a couple of cocktails, and if she drank two cups of coffee she lost practically all control of herself and was not accountable for her actions, her hilarity approaching that of alcoholic intoxication.

Nervousness and insanity: The nervous decadence of the present-day civilized races is certainly due to their excessive indulgence in tea and coffee. It is an actual fact that a surprisingly large percentage of the insanity cases in England and Ireland, where tea is the national drink, are traced directly to inordinate tea consumption.

What specialists say: Chas. B. Towns, a specialist in the treatment of drug addicts, says that of all the various addicts who come under his jurisdiction for treatment, he has round the genuine dyed-in-the-wool caffeine habitué worst of all and more intractable than the cocaine fiend.

Herbert Hutchinson, M. D., clinical lecturer on Neurology and Psychiatry at the University of Maryland, states that "Coffee intoxication is a disease which is probably more common than is generally supposed—the profession not alive to its symptoms, as it has not yet penetrated into the classics of pathology and hygiene. The most pronounced and tenacious factor of coffee intoxication is tremor, occurring in at least 60% of the cases and often persisting many weeks after the disuse of coffee."

Dr. Geo. M. Miles of Atlanta, Ga., Professor of Physiology in Southern College of Pharmacy, says: "Coffee is a drug, no matter under what flag it sails, and it tends to induce a drug habit just as does any other stimulant."

Dr. Emil King in an article on "Tea and Coffee Intoxication" asserts that "both tea and coffee contain relatively a large proportion of active ingredients, and we may be surprised that we do not meet even more cases of poisoning. I feel certain that the causes of poisonous action by tea and coffee are relatively frequent and that they are often overlooked. Constant over-stimulation of the brain leads to exhaustion, insomnia, vertigo, headache, neuralgia, flashes of light, mental dullness with exhaustion of mind, disinclination to work and melancholia with apprehension of evil."

Dr. James Wood, reporting 100 cases of coffee poison, says: "Of these 100 cases, 20% complained of persistent dizziness, 19% of indigestion, 45% of headache, 20% of despondency, 19% of palpitation of the heart and 15% of insomnia."

Dr. Wm. H. Leszyinsky, consulting neurologist of the Manhattan Eye and Ear Hospital, observes that 'The habitual daily indulgence in coffee, even in moderate quantity, by those who are over-sensitive to its action, invariably leads to persistent functional disorder of the nervous system, as well as to a disturbance in digestion. These rapidly subside when coffee is discontinued. These patients usually complain of general headaches, nervousness, apprehension in regard to some unknown impending trouble, mental depression, irritability, insomnia or restless sleep, bad dreams, sudden starting in sleep, awakening in profuse perspiration, occasional or frequent vertigo, general tremulousness, diminishing muscular power, precordial depression (feeling of smothering around the heart), palpitation, loss of appetite, frequent eructations of gas and constipation.'"

So from this general resume by noteworthy physicians it would not seem that coffee and tea were such harmless drinks after all. Their ultimate effects are comparable to those of alcohol and tobacco, although the prohibitionist, who sees pale melancholy and red ruin in a glass of wine, would regard you as slightly demented if you suggested that he was getting very similar effects from his daily coffee. Neither would the fervent member of the anti-cigarette league rank you with the cognoscenti if you confided to him that he got the same kick out of his morning cup of coffee that the smoker derived from his Camel or Lucky Strike.

Remember, I do not smoke. Neither do I drink tea, coffee or alcoholic stimulants. I have done all these things to excess in past years, and I know their effects. I merely wish to point out how the short sighted, narrow-minded reformer can go along vindictively pointing out the mote in his neighbor's eye when the beam in his own eye is so large that it is a miracle his sight is not wholly obstructed.

SALT

I teach you how to live — you decide how to die. — Estes.

Despite the progress of science, the correction of dietetic errors and the various advanced methods of treatment for disease, sickness and death pursue their relentless path from month to month and year to year. Although exhaustive research on bacteria has proved effective to a great extent in coping with many diseases, it has been futile in the handling of maladies of baffling character, and now the attention of medical science has been directed to the enemy within the walls of the fortress. The keen eye of the medical profession looks askance upon sodium chloride, the accessory of every table, and this hapless condiment salt, is charged with treason. A traitor to health, instead of an agent of, it is to be banished from the table completely.

The diseases and poisons resulting from the excessive use of salt afford enough material for countless books to be written on the subject. You need no salt whatever in a diet of *natural* foods. The human system requires only about 15 grains per day of sodium chloride, yet the quantity taken by the average person is from 200 to 500 grains each day. Uncooked vegetables and fresh fruits contain sufficient of the natural salts, including sodium chloride, to meet the requirements of the body. Of course, when these vegetables and fruits are cooked, the mineral salts are drained off with the water into the sink; consequently some of the salts must be artificially restored to make the foods at all palatable.

Salt is a powerful irritant which stimulates the entire system and acts directly upon the organs of generation, inciting the sex impulses. Where this condition is persistent the over-functioning of the sex organs is the result, and disease and general depletion can only follow.

Salt contracts the muscles of the uterus and destroys their flexibility and elasticity. This is one of the reasons why *Caesarian* operations are a necessity in many cases. When salt has been dispensed with entirety, there will not be the heavy congestion and general tension in the pelvic and uterine region; the tissues will be soft and flexible, and a normal, natural birth without laceration will be achieved.

Research proves that salt is responsible for cancer. Experiments and profound study of the subject have disclosed the fact that *cancer* is a disease of civilization and is not found among tribes of savage people. Practically the only notable contrast between the foods of civilized and savage peoples is the addition of sodium chloride, or table salt, to the diet of civilization. Formerly cancer was a rare disease, but as the production of salt has increased in proportion to the demand, cancer has become more and more prevalent. Another startling fact is that cancer does not originate as a malignant growth, but is a simple, benign tumor which, due to persistent irritation and the inability of the bloodstream to heal, eventually passes into a malignant state —and proves fatal.

No cell of the body can become cancerous through its own independent action but must receive its irritating incentive from the chemical composition of the plasma (the fluid content of the blood), an agent of which is sodium chloride.

Medical science goes on to tell us that there must be an idiosyncrasy to salt in persons developing cancer. Thus, not all salt eaters develop cancer, but all cancerous people are salt eaters.

Sodium and potassium are both elements in cell life, but sodium is found in greater quantities in the secretions and fluids of the body, whereas potassium exists in a greater degree as an ingredient in the cell. The equal distribution of these two elements in the cell constitutes a healthy cell. Hence, if a superfluous amount of sodium is taken into the body, the potassium element is crowded out, and although potassium is the rightful ingredient, the sodium displaces it and becomes the predominating element of the cell. Naturally the cell will try to eliminate an irritating substance, and then begins the first local inflammation.

Cancer is not a communicable disease and cannot be transmitted through hereditary influences. However, the idiosyncrasy to salt in the parent can be transmitted to the child, making it liable to a cancerous development.

Cancerous cases put upon a saltless diet and treated with administrations of potassium nitrate, which restores this missing element to the cell, have responded immediately to treatment and have been effectively cured.

Extensive inquiry has failed to disclose the authenticity of the generally-accepted report that all animals must have salt or they will perish. No one has ever witnessed the pilgrimage of animals to the natural salt springs, or "licks." Deer frequently, at certain seasons, do resort to brine springs, but it is only a tradition that buffalo follow suit. Moreover, in these salt springs are found large amounts of lime, iron, sulphur and other minerals. As one authority has suggested, it is reasonable to assume that the wild animals may crave and seek at these springs certain minerals which nature deprives them of at that particular time of the year. Horses and cows of civilization are fed salt, but a block of the coarse salt used for this purpose lasts the animal many months. It is an artificial taste, and some horses and cows refuse salt when given it.   Birds avoid it.   It is fatal to chickens.

Why does man eat what animals are intelligent enough to reject.

One cancer specialist who is waging relentless war against the use of table salt, cites the case of a pet cat which was brought to him for treatment of a cancerous lip. Convinced of the popular fallacy that all animals must have salt, the owner had liberally seasoned the cat's food with salt from the time it was a small kitten until it was about three and one-half years of age, at which time it developed cancer of the lip. The cat became sick and refused food and lost its fur. Given treatment for cancer precisely as a human patient, the cat was cured and a new coat of fur grown. Those who are worried over falling hair and imminent baldness should give this fact consideration. The cat's fur fell out—it was ill and developed cancer when fed on salt. The salt was omitted from its food, the cancer cured and a new coat of fur was grown. Draw your own conclusions.

The human bloodstream contains three parts of sodium chloride to one thousand parts.

Salt is eliminated principally through the kidneys and skin. Statistics show that the average person consumes about two-thirds of an ounce of salt daily. About one-eighth is lost through the skin, and the greater part of the remainder is eliminated through the kidneys. Observation proves that salt disappears entirely from the urine when wasting is prolonged.

Dropsy is produced, in the majority of cases, by the accumulation of salt in the tissues—the kidneys are unable to eliminate the excess of salt, and as it is pushed out into the tissues it must, of course, be held in solution by water. For every half ounce of salt retained in the body, a pound of water will be retained to hold it in solution. Hence it will be easily understood why the weight increases in dropsy, Bright's disease and edema.

Observation also shows that the kidneys fail to eliminate salt at the usual rate in various other diseases, including pneumonia, pleurisy, typhoid fever, jaundice, cirrhosis of the liver, smallpox and some forms of heart disease.

In extreme cases it has been observed that complete retention of salt preceded immediate death. Specimens of urine of patients suffering moderately from diabetes showed no sodium chloride whatever, although some was being taken in the food. Repeated examinations within twenty-four hours showed no trace of salt. At the end of the second day the patient was dead. There had been no previous symptoms of a serious condition. Other cases similar to this are on record showing in all instances that the complete retention of salt was fatal.

One two-hundredth of its weight in salt administered to a dog will cause convulsions and death.

A case was reported of a young woman whose death was induced by a half-pound dose of salt taken as a vermifuge.

Postmortems performed after deaths due to overdoses of salt have led to the conclusions that the excessive use of salt causes chronic kidney disease, as these postmortems reveal enlargement and heavy degeneration of the kidneys.

Practically no chemical change in salt is made by the cells of the body. In other words, the composition of salt remains unalterable, and if more salt is eaten than can be eliminated, the excess accumulates in the cellular walls, and subsequent irritation begins.

To people who have always been heavy salt-eaters, this anti-salt propaganda will come as a sensationally-new fad to be dismissed with a shrug. However, it is not new. The medical profession of the British Isles became involved in such a heated controversy in the latter part of the 19th century that the fraternity split into two factions—the Salts and the Anti-Salts. At this time, the leader of the anti-salt faction issued the statement that he would advise alcoholic drinks and vinegar in preference to the constant use of salt.

Salt was known to the ancients as a corrosive poison. The sages and philosophers of the early centuries knew of the injuries man incurred through the use of salt, and warnings against this indulgence were carved on tablets of stone.

Stefannsson, the explorer, in his narrative of experiences with the white Eskimos, stated that they had never tasted salt until he and his followers went among them. The Eskimo's aversion to salt was very strong. To safeguard his meat supply Stefannsson had only to sprinkle it liberally with salt, and the light-fingered natives of the Polar region left it severely alone.

Dr. Harris Houghton of New York City, a writer and lecturer on pathological subjects, has demonstrated that salt is very dangerous to people with high blood pressure. He states that 80% of the *high blood pressure* cases can be promptly relieved by a carefully-administered saltless diet. Specialists in the treatment of diabetes and physicians famous for research in blood chemistry support Dr. Houghton in this saltless diet for blood-pressure cases.

Some conditions of extremely white skin are attributed to the destructive action of salt on the capillary circulation. Florid complexions, tendency to nose-bleed and a feeling of tension in the head constitute what is termed plethora, another symptom which is evidenced in cases of excessive salt eating. Still another symptom is progressive wasting and emaciation, especially in young children, where there is no obvious or ascertainable cause.

Salt throat, where the throat is more or less sore and streaked alternately with red and white, red circles on the fingers back of the nails (being a more pronounced color at this point than on other parts of the hand), and dandruff are all manifestations of a system crowded with sodium chloride.

It is a grave mistake to permit children to eat salt freely on such foods as celery, onions, radishes, etc. Some parents will even give the children salt in the palm of the hand when they seem to relish it. Neither children nor adults should have any salt added to their food, much less eat it plentifully as though it were a sweet. If parents realized that habits of early masturbation in children were a direct result of the eating of salty foods, they would be very guarded about the children's diet Salt produces an irritation in the genital organs, which causes the child to scratch itself. As this continues, the irritation is apt to develop unwholesome desires in the child and lead him into habits which are ruinous to his mental and physical growth.

Cancer, hardening of the arteries, impaired vision, defective hearing, dizziness and insomnia are only a few of the many dangerous and chronic ailments which may be traced to cumulative salt poisoning.

Extreme sensibility to pain, undue irritability of the nerves, melancholia and many forms of sex perversion and abnormalities are direct results of the excessive use of sodium chloride.

Reformers rant and churches decry the social evils of the day, but if they would bend their energies toward spreading the gospel of pure, unadulterated, wholesome food, more would be accomplished in a few years than they will achieve in a century with their sermons on morality and abstinence.

Human beings are not basically immoral. They are victims of formidable enemies in the guise of highly-seasoned, irritating foods. With systems daily saturated with a mineral which acts directly upon the delicate and easily-aroused sex organs, the normal sex desires are so increased as to become an obsession which leads to abnormality and perversion and eventual insanity.

The accompanying article, taken from the *Chicago Tribune* of Oct. 15, 1922, illustrates the present degenerate condition of the human race. When we have reached a point where premature weakness and debility of the generative organs, through high living and loose morals, necessitates the abduction of unsuspecting individuals for the removal of their vital glands which are to be used in restoring lost vigor and health to a man whose purse is large enough to conceal the dastardly theft and protect the perpetrators thereof, then perhaps the world will awaken to its peril and, throwing off its indifference, will seek earnestly for the source of danger. That this source may be found on the dining table of every home and restaurant will come as a startling announcement to a salt-soaked world but not to the studious medical scientists who have been poring over dull facts for years and tirelessly experimenting on stubborn ailments of malignant character.

COMB CITY IN HUNT FOR GLAND THIEF
Medical Society Aids Search for Doctor
Involved in the Operation.

SECOND VICTIM REPORTED
Lured Into Taxicab; Hospitals Yield No Clue Nor Is
Companion Found.

Hunt for a surgeon who carried through the first human gland theft in history was under way by the Chicago police today.

At the same time, Dr. H. M. McKechnie, president of the Chicago Medical Society, announced that his organization would do everything in its power to aid the police.

The victim of the gland theft was Joseph Wozniak, a laborer, who came here recently from the Wisconsin beet fields.

According to the story Wozniak told Dr. A. Sampolinski, who reported the case to the police, he was walking along a street when an automobile drew up; four men leaped out, threw a bag over his head and dragged him into the machine.

Expert Performs Operation.

He was chloroformed, he said, and when he regained consciousness he found himself on a sidewalk under aviaduct. The operation had been performed—with expert skill.

It was believed by the police that some wealthy and perhaps aged man has benefited by the criminal action.

Wozniak is 34 years old, has been married twelve years, but has no children.

Police believe there also may have been an operation performed on Wozniak's companion at the time, who has not been located.

According to Wozniak, he and a man named Kuchnisky, or Pruchnicki, living in the vicinity of Milwaukee Avenue and Robey Street, set out Wednesday afternoon "to get so drunk they would have to be carried home." They later met the gland bandits who abducted Wozniak, he says, and chloroformed him.

That the men also took Wozniak's companion and performed a similar operation on him is the belief of Capt. Thomas Caughlin of the Marquette station.

May Have Been Lured

There are other theories that the police are working on, too. One is that Wozniak might have been lured into the hands of the gland pirates by the companion. The other is that he might have willingly parted with his gland for a sum of money as he has been out of work. But an investigation by the police failed to reveal that the man had had any extra money recently.

The surgeon who performed the operation is unknown to the medical profession, but physicians throughout the city banded together today to ferret him out and drive him from the city.

The man who became the victim of the operation robbery is under the care of Dr. A. S. Sampolinski.

"Outrage" Doctors Say.

"Outrage is too alight a word to characterize this doctor's action," Dr. McKechnie said. "Our society will do everything in our power to bring this man to justice. No surgeon worthy of the name would have resorted to any such disgraceful and criminal conduct."

Dr. Max Thorek, associated with Dr. Serge Voronoff of Paris in the original demonstrations of the value of glandular transplantations, expressed the hope that the surgeon responsible for the theft of Wozniak's gland might suffer a fate like that which "his money-mania had caused him to inflict."

Wozniak, who lives at 1857 W. Seventeenth Street, had been out of work since returning to America after fighting in the world war for America and, later, in the battle for Poland's independence. Last Wednesday he set out to find a job.

"Early in the afternoon I met a man at Milwaukee Avenue and Noble Street," he told in an earlier account. "He listened to my story of how I had sought a job in vain, lent me $10 and bought me a number of drinks. Finally, he said he would order a taxicab and have me driven home.

"The cab came and he steered me into it. Inside were four men. I had not time to look them over because I was slugged and a cone was put over my mouth and nose."

Awakens in Vacant Lot

The man was taken, evidently, to a hospital, because the knife wound as examined later by Dr. Sampolinski demonstrated that the operation had been performed by an expert. Thursday morning Wozniak awakened in a vacant lot.

"I did not know that I had been operated on," he said. "I went home thinking I had been drunk, but I had the taste of ether or chloroform in my mouth. I felt intense pain and called Dr. Sampolinski, who found out the truth."

It is almost impossible not to eat some salt, particularly if many meals are eaten in a restaurant. Breads carry salt as well as butter and cheese. Sweet butter, however, may be obtained in many restaurants and is most delicious.

Salted butter contains 30 grains of salt to the ounce, which totals 480 grains to the pound. The average person eats at least two to three ounces of butter a day. Some eat much more.   In this one article of food alone, from 60 to 90 grains of salt are taken into the body, to say nothing of the other foods containing salt.

Once you have become accustomed to a salt-less diet, you will soon become very sensitive to the action of salt, and where you formerly ate salted meats and fish with great relish, you will find that they are not so palatable and leave the membranes of the throat and mouth dry and irritated.

If you want HEALTH, omit all salted foods and break yourself of the salt habit.

ALCOHOL

"Man, by his imprudence in diet and drink and other manifold excesses, lives only one-quarter his allotted time."

Prohibition has limited the public sale of alcoholic drinks, but it has in no way restricted the private use of them. Men and women who never drank before the 18th Amendment was passed have since cultivated a taste for alcohol and have considered it an obligation to violate the law in retaliation for the restrictions placed upon their personal liberty.

Accounts of deaths due to the effects of home-brew and spurious concoctions containing denatured alcohol, ether, formaldehyde and even chloroform are to be found in papers every day. To satisfy the craze for drink, the alcohol addicts resort to any and all substitutes for whiskey, beer and wine.

The effects of the alcoholic drinks sold before prohibition were serious enough but many of the home brews and cheap concoctions stealthily peddled about are fatal and disastrous; even moderate use of alcoholic drinks of the purest kind produces conditions which lead to an early death.

High blood pressure, hardening of the arteries, hob-nailed liver, alcoholic heart and Bright's disease are brought on by the use of alcohol.

Alcohol over-stimulates the entire body at first and after its effects have worn off, the reaction is a loss of vitality of the nerves and tissues and a general depleted condition of the system. Alcohol eats out the mucous membrane which lines the stomach, and impaired digestion, dyspepsia and cancer are among the many complications which follow.

Alcohol has an immediate effect on the kidneys, causing them to over-function.

It has a highly simulative effect on the sex organs and a subsequent reaction which often impairs the normal sex functions entirely.

The over-functioning of any part of the body eventually results in the loss of activity to that part.

Alcohol affects all parts of the body and consequently the general health is affected.

Excessive use of alcohol leads to insanity, blindness, loss of hair and teeth, paresis, locomotor-ataxia, apoplexy, paralysis, et cetera.

The body, if fed on proper foods, generates its own alcohol in quantities sufficient to meet the requirements and afford the necessary stimulation. The system derives enough sodium chloride or salt from the foods, if eaten in the raw natural state and the commercial salt taken into the body forms an excess which is highly irritating and provocative of disease.

So also does the manufactured alcohol menace the health and life when taken into the body. Alcohol generated from cooked foods in the body, paralyzes. Alcohol generated from Raw Foods in the body, stimulates.

Those who desire health, happiness and long life should shun alcohol in all its forms.

TOBACCO

Because of the universal use and the subtle deception of its insidious effects, tobacco has not been branded as definitely as its criminal cohort, alcohol. A lax, indifferent air of toleration is granted the tobacco user—the habit is generally accepted, and as long as the tobacco habitué confines himself to cigars, cigarettes and pipes and does not resort to chewing the weed, he is admitted to the best circles and regarded as a man of mild habits. Let him so far forget himself, however, as to *chew* tobacco, and a different story is heard. The hue and cry sent up denounces him as a filthy creature to be shunned by all. Yet, only because the chewing of tobacco is so obvious, so obnoxious, does it bring down scathing censure upon its user's head. The evils of and injuries due to smoking are so numerous as to seem incredible, and when they are enumerated to the inveterate smoker, he smiles knowingly and mentally registers you as a nut. No smoker will ever admit that he suffers to any degree from his habit. He will always attribute any ailment he is afflicted with to almost any other cause than tobacco, even though it is a disorder which even a layman can diagnose as a result of smoking.

The consumption of tobacco in 1920 averaged 180 ounces per capita, and in that same year 62,000,000,000 cigarettes were manufactured, 46,000,000,000 of which were consumed in this country—averaging 460 cigarettes for every man, woman and child.

Nicotine—which ranks second only to prussic acid as a deadly poison—is only one of the many virulent poisons found in the tobacco leaf. Nicotine is considered by experts the most insidious and life-shortening of all, however. Pyridine, collidine, carbon monoxide, furfurole and ammonia are a few of the others. All animals rapidly succumb to nicotine poisoning, regardless of how it is administered—

whether by the intestinal canal, subcutaneously or in a wound. The animal is soon overcome, falls into severe convulsions and dies.

Pyridine is one of the poisons used to denature alcohol and render it unfit for internal use.

Furfurole, an aldehyde, belongs to the alcohol group and is the poison in tobacco which is responsible for the nervous tremor and twitching which is characteristic of the cigarette addict. Its presence in cigarettes and cigars is due to the burning of glycerine, which, in combination with saltpetre, is blended with the tobacco to preserve the quality of the cigarette for a "good smoke." Furfurole is a component part of fusel oil, and it is also one of the basic agents found in improperly aged whiskey. Authorities state that one cigarette may contain as much furfurole as two or three ounces of bad whiskey. Furfurole is an extremely dangerous poison, 50 times as poisonous as alcohol. Small doses produce irritation—large doses cause convulsions and epilepsy.

Collidine is a fluid possessing a very penetrating odor, and it is this poison which is the principal factor in giving the pungent odor to tobacco. It is a poisonous alkaloid, the 20th part of a drop of which will kill a frog. Le Bon, who isolated collidine, has demonstrated that the breathing of this poison will produce muscular feebleness and vertigo.

The man who lights a cigar, smokes awhile and lets the cigar die out and relights it, after having kept it in his mouth, chewing the end while he talked and breathed, little realizes that he is thereby creating the dangerous carbon monoxide gas, the same gas which is contained in the evil-smelling fumes expelled through the exhaust of an automobile, and which yearly takes a large toll in deaths when workers in small garages tinker with their cars, keeping the exhaust open and the doors of the garage closed. Numbness and suffocation come on very suddenly and overcome the worker before he is able to get into fresh air. The smoker, by holding the cigar in his mouth when he talks and breathes, allows the saliva to run along the filler, dampening the inside of the cigar. The imperfect combustion results in the production of carbon monoxide, which is a highly active blood poison. It destroys the red cells of the blood and prevents their absorbing oxygen, which is so essential for life.

Acrolein is a poison which is found in the smoke of burning paper. It is a great irritant and has a violent action on the nerve centers, producing mental degeneracy, which makes particularly rapid progress among adolescents. Edison has stated that he considers this degeneracy permanent and incurable. These poisons are all generated as a result of burning the tobacco, and they are almost parallel to nicotine itself as regards their dangerous effects.

There has always been the much-mooted question as to whether or not cigarettes are doped. Formerly opium was employed in the manufacture of some of the oriental brands of smokes, which produced such a subtle, soothing effect. However, since the passing of the anti-narcotic law, manufacturers have been obliged to content themselves with essential oils, extracts and concentrated essences to lend a distinctive flavor to their products.

Evils of pipe-smoking: Many men think they escape the graver effects of tobacco by smoking a pipe instead of cigarettes and cigars, and yet experiments have proven that the liquid essence contained in a pipe after a man has been smoking a few hours, is almost pure nicotine and is strong enough to kill an insect or any small bird or animal within a few minutes. One *cigar* contains enough *nicotine* to kill a man if the entire quantity were taken internally.

The erroneous idea that tobacco is healthful: The facts about tobacco have been so carefully repressed and so successfully distorted that many smokers contend their health is improved through its use. Although frequently we hear of some hardy old chap who has reached the century mark, or passed it, who ascribes his ruggedness to a beloved pipe or a favorite brand of chewing tobacco, no actual proof of tobacco's merits has ever been set forth. It is not uncommon to hear of another centenarian who attributes his longevity to a wicked brand of hard liquor. It is a freak of nature that these steady smokers and inebriates do live to a very mature age occasionally, but close investigation generally has revealed that they are mountaineers or farmers who have led active lives, engaged in strenuous labor and were out of doors constantly, thus deriving strength and resistance to throw off the poisons injected into their systems through tobacco and whiskey. These individuals have also often inherited a predisposition to long lives. Coming from the stock which produced the rugged pioneer type, a man with such powerful antecedents might live 150 years if he had not acquired habits which slowly undermined his great resistance.

Since the passing of the 18th Amendment, the prohibitionists must be disappointed to find that not all the evils of the world have been rooted out. Indeed the impression that tobacco is as injurious as alcoholic stimulants is daily gaining ground, and not only physicians and specialists are carefully experimenting with it, but business men employing large numbers of workers in various branches of industry are studiously computing the effects of tobacco upon the efficiency of their employees, and the man who does not use it obtains a preference over the smoker.

All criminals smokers: It is a well known fact that the history of almost any criminal discloses the fact that he is an inveterate smoker. He learns to smoke when he is young and drifts to pool rooms, where he smokes and passes the time. Later he strays to saloons, falls in with bad companions and eventually develops the criminal instinct.

Gunmen, gangsters and prostitutes, without exception, are excessive cigarette smokers.

Tobacco, and particularly in the form of cigarettes, is a source of protoplasmic poisoning and causes *degenerative disorders of the brain,* heart, blood vessels and kidneys. Toxins in tobacco destroy the elasticity of the blood vessels and cause an increased tension. This in turn places a strain on the liver, kidneys and the other vital organs whose perfect activity is necessary to keep the blood free from poisons. The inhaling of a cigarette arrests oxygenation and inhibits the natural carrying off of poisons, since the blood's purification depends upon oxygenation of the lungs.

Tobacco stunts growth: Tobacco hinders the growth and development of the young by thwarting the functions of the nervous system. It impairs the digestion, and thus, by interfering with perfect assimilation, it causes malnutrition and is responsible for the stunted physique and sluggish brain of the youthful smoker.

Tobacco heart is not generally viewed with alarm, but it is a condition which is often extremely serious, and a decrease in the use of tobacco or a complete abstinence may restore the heart to a nearly, if not completely, normal condition. Death may occur as a result of a sudden shock or unusual strain in the meantime.

Acid dyspepsia, catarrhal conditions of nose and throat and ear—even blindness—follow the excessive indulgence of tobacco. Due to the breaking down of the nervous system, with subsequent mental degeneration, insanity is frequently due to slow nicotine poison.

Reaction of nicotine: Nicotine first stimulates and afterwards paralyzes the motor nerves of the involuntary muscles and the secreting nerves of the glands, also the spinal cord. It contracts the pupils of the eyes, slows and depresses the heart, first lowers and then raises the arterial tension and reduces the body temperature. *Death* has occurred from a toxic dose of *nicotine* within *three minutes,* the only symptoms being a wild stare and a deep sigh.

The man who claims that his brain functions more clearly and that his thoughts run more freely under the stimulus of a good smoke is merely reacting to the drug the same as any other dope fiend. It is yet to be proved that any sound, healthy man thinks better under the influence of tobacco than he does without. Experiments with nicotine extracts and *inhalations* of tobacco on animals have produced hardening of the arteries. Observation shows that practically the same condition is brought about in men and women.

Effects on efficiency: That muscular precision and clarity of thought are seriously impaired by the use of tobacco was demonstrated some time ago when the International Commission of the Young Men's Christian Association of New York City made experiments on young men between 21 and 25 who were being trained as physical directors and were in excellent condition. Smokers and non-smokers were put to the same tests to determine the effects on both. Both were put through the tests first without a smoke and then after a smoke. A single cigar or cigarette was generally used. The first experiment was a test of the heart action and blood pressure after the smoking of one cigar. In all cases the heart was so disturbed that it took considerable time to return to normal, and the blood pressure also was greatly increased. The second experiment was given a year later and proved conclusively that smokers have a higher heart rate than non-smokers and that the return to normal after exercise was greatly delayed after smoking. To illustrate: In 94 out of 118 smoking tests, 62.72 per cent, the heart rate was increased and did not return to normal in 15 minutes. In 72 out of 74 tests in which the men did not smoke, fully 97 per cent did return to normal in less than 15 minutes, the average being only five minutes. The smoker does not become fully habituated to smoking. Tests in muscular precision followed. The men were required to draw lines with a pen on a chart between narrow columns. Every time the sides were touched an error was registered. To test the co-ordination of the large muscles, the men were required to lunge at a target with a fencing foil. In both tests all the men showed a loss in precision, proving conclusively that even one or two cigars (which were used in the tests) had a very decided effect.

Three tests for accuracy were given. In these tests they were required to pitch an official baseball. In Test A, after the men had smoked one cigar, there was a 12 per cent loss in accuracy. In Test B, after smoking two cigars, the scores showed a 14.5 % per cent loss. In the *final* Test C, no cigars were smoked, and a 30-minute rest was taken instead. A 9 per cent increase in accuracy was the result.

College and school teachers, psychologists, clinicians and efficiency experts are unanimous in their condemnation of tobacco. It is not used as a medicine and not even listed in the U. S. Pharmacopia as a remedy for disease.

Cancer of the tongue is more frequent among men than women, and particularly in the United States—only 2 per cent of the cases being women, so it seems perfectly reasonable to attribute its cause, at least partly, to the use of tobacco. *Cancer* of the tongue is occasionally found in a non-smoker, but it is very rare and due to some exciting cause which is a local and long-continued irritation, such as neglected teeth, the use of clay pipes, which are dry and irritating to the mouth, salivary deposits, bridge work and artificial plates. General Grant was an inveterate smoker, and it was said that he held a cigar in his mouth from the time he arose until he retired. He died of cancer of the tongue as a result of tobacco irritation. Ex-Kaiser Wilhelm's father was also a victim of *cancer* of the tongue, due to the use of tobacco. Of 550 deaths in England due to cancer of the tongue, 447 of these cases were men and only 73 were women. In the order of their facility to produce irritation, the following are listed: Tobacco, jagged teeth, poorly-fitting artificial teeth, salivary calculus, sharp pipe stems, cigar and cigarette holders and chemical caustics. An eminent head surgeon states that one of the greatest errors in medical treatment is the application of severe caustics to simple sores, as it seems to have a tendency to induce a chronic condition which may develop a malignant character.

A sensational case of cancer of the tongue attracted wide attention a number of years ago when Dr. Nicholas Senn, the famous surgeon, now dead, operated on the patient and removed his tongue. Much publicity was given the man who was willing to take one chance in a million to save his life, even though he would never speak again if he did survive. He was doomed to die a painful death by slow torture if the cancerous condition were permitted to go on and he stood a slight chance of living if his tongue were removed. He was feted and banqueted by his friends up until a few hours before the operation. His tongue was removed, he left the hospital after a time and resumed his affairs, but the shock to the system was apparently too great to be surmounted, for he died shortly afterward.

THE CANCEROUS TONGUE WAS DUE TO THE USE OF TOBACCO!

Habit difficult to check: In order to stamp out the evils of the tobacco habit, it will be necessary to organize against it just as it was necessary to organize against alcohol. Since the effects of tobacco are equally as serious as those of alcohol, but less rapid in their culmination, it is not recognized as a dangerous poison, but, like the traditional wolf, it stalks about in sheep's clothing. Since the habit seems to be one which constantly grows and once acquired, is difficult to check, it were easier not to contract it at all. Relative to checking the habit, once it is contracted, observation indicates that tobacco weakens a man's will, even as other dope, so that if the desire to decrease its use is there, the individual seems helpless and unable to resist the lure of the cigarette, cigar or pipe which brings him drowsy comfort and surcease from thought.

The author was a habitual smoker for about thirty years and so has had a slight experience and not all of his knowledge is gained from observation. He averaged some 50 cigarettes a day, and after finally giving up cigarette smoking, he comforted himself with about 25 cigars daily. He feels fully conversant with the effects of tobacco upon the throat and mucous membranes of the head. The constant use of tobacco causes dryness of the membranes, irritation and a tight, hacking and gagging cough. As has been stated, inhaling prevents oxygenation of the lungs, and this is why excessive cigarette smokers develop *tuberculosis*. Asthma, tonsil trouble, nervous twitching of eyes and muscles and various forms of irritability are among the evil effects resulting from the habitual use of tobacco.

Stomach disorders due to smoking: Some time ago there was an article in Physical Culture Magazine by a man who had suffered for years with extreme heartburn. Fie had not smoked until he entered college, and, falling in line with the habits of his fellow students, he learned to smoke, not wisely, but too well. According to his own accounts, he smoked cigarettes, then cigars, stogies, a pipe and finally, as a crowning achievement to grace his various accomplishments, he learned the delicate art of using snuff and chewing tobacco. After this had gone on for some time he became a victim of a number of ailments, the most pronounced and painful of which was heartburn. To relieve this he took quantities of baking soda. Physicians diagnosed his case—advised operations for gall-stones and stomach ulcer. One friend told him that his stomach had at some time become stretched from over-eating and this was responsible for the pain he felt when the stomach was not distended. He dodged operations and treated with a chiropractor, who helped him, but he was obliged to continue with his doses of soda. During his wanderings he finally fell into the hands of a physician who treated him for stomach ulcer and gave him bismuth and silver nitrate. This treatment covered a period of 18 months, at the end of which time the pigmentation of his skin was changed (a condition which is now permanent, he states), and the "ulcer" continued gaily on its way, still uncured. After about seventeen years of this misdirected treatment, the man in question was finally taken by his brother to an expert diagnostician. This diagnostician examined him minutely — carefully, to the last detail—and at the conclusion of the examination pronounced him "a damn fool." (I quote him.) He then told the sufferer that he had no stomach ulcer whatever; that he required no operation. The doctor summed up the trouble by informing him that he smoked too much—explained that there is a certain ganglion of nerves particularly susceptible to nicotine and when they become irritated the stomach is supplied with an excess acid which causes heartburn and digestive discomfort. Thus the soda relieved him temporarily by solidifying the acid. Likewise a full stomach dilutes the acid and ameliorates the pain. The physician informed him that tobacco was a rank poison and that he would be cured at once by discontinuing his use of it.

The patient was much amused, for the diagnosis was rendered between puffs of cigarettes and clouds of smoke. The physician, however, explained that while he himself smoked a great deal he was affected very slightly, although he admitted that he would probably be a better doctor if he didn't smoke at all.

The sufferer from heartburn was sufficiently impressed with the lecture to stop smoking at once. He was cured in two days. He confesses that he occasionally slips and reverts to his old habit of smoking, only to suffer intensely with heartburn, which nothing will cure but complete abstinence from tobacco. As he himself states, it is hard to understand that phase of human nature which will make a man go back to a habit which he knows is bad for him and which causes acute discomfort.

Tobacco habit generally disagreeable: Aside from the physical injuries due to the persistent use of tobacco, the habit is a nasty, offensive one. The teeth of the smoker become stained and discolored; the breath reeks of stagnant smoke even when the smoker is not indulging; his fingers are usually stained; his hair and clothes are saturated with the fumes of tobacco, and although the individual may be scrupulously clean about his person, he is constantly enveloped with a disagreeable, noxious odor which is distasteful to people of refined and delicate sensibilities.

The present day period of flappers and cake-eaters, an epoch in the evolution of twentieth century Youth, is responsible for the lowered vitality and resistance of young men and women. These dashing, sophisticated infants who cultivate the habits of smoking and drinking as assiduously as our grandmothers learned to cook and knit, should be stripped, the girls of their filmy hose and gossamer gowns, the boys of their pinch-back coats and patent leather dancing pumps, given a good, old-fashioned thrashing and started upon the road to sane living instead of being permitted to hurl their youth, strength and morals upon the rocks of pernicious and popular custom.

That these fast habits of smoking and drinking breed degeneracy and immorality is evinced by the brazen actions and nonchalant regard for the proprieties, not only characteristic of the youthful element which frequents public dance-halls and restaurants but even of the sons and daughters of cultured, wealthy families. The flappers vie with each other in their attempts to be sensational. The thinner her hose, the lower the neck of the gown, the more exaggerated her general effect, the more striking and popular is the girl. To create an impression of wit, wisdom and smartness, she drinks cocktails and "hooch," refers familiarly to "something on the hip," and takes up cigarette smoking as a matter of course. She learns to inhale, not because she really enjoys it but just to show that she is complete master of the art and because she thinks it is the correct thing to do. Thus a practice begun purely for effect soon becomes a habit and before long the girl is hopelessly addicted to cigarettes.

The young, pimply-faced striplings who are contemptuously designated as flappers, cake-eaters, lounge lizards, bench-bunnies and tea-hounds, are appalling spectacles to look upon as future citizens and fathers and possible national and civic leaders.

With their flat chests, "S" like spines, lanky, scrawny, under-developed bodies consumed by the fires of alcohol and the deadly poisons of tobacco, they gaze with patronizing eyes and smirking face upon any man, the cut of whose clothes is not quite the last word and whose cravat may not be the most ultra thing for the true man about town, and if his collar is more than an inch wide and his hair not greased to just the proper mode, Heaven help him, for he is socially doomed, an outcast not to be admitted within the pale of the so-called smart set.

These callow youths are devoid of character, brains, morals and ability. With rare exceptions they are inveterate smokers. Their bodies are weak and puny, poisoned with tobacco. Their lungs are constricted, under-developed, and in many cases atrophied and diseased. Their mentality is a minus quantity. They are neither men nor women but poison-soaked nonentities, stalking the earth with a misconceived idea of their own importance.

It is pitiable to see them, both sexes, lounging around the theatres, hotels and cafes, languidly puffing a cigarette, girls as well as boys; the female novice's awkwardness sharply contrasted by the perfect poise of the "old-timer."

The frivolous flapper is ignorant and not to be entirely condemned if she imitates the vicious example set by her more mature sisters who have apparently taken leave of their senses in favor of the fads which will wreck their nerves and destroy their health.

The use of tobacco is a crime! Its effects on the lungs alone should be sufficient to damn it for all mankind. It is responsible for loss of memory, sluggish skin, pallor, warped ideas, perverted impulses and, above all of the lesser evils, for the degenerate mental condition wherein the smoker is impressed with his or her superiority to all those with whom he or she comes in contact excepting the members of the "klan."

With these conditions becoming more and more prevalent day by day, can anyone deny that smoking is a deadly evil, which is paralyzing the finer instincts and obscuring the higher motives of our children?

Its demoralizing effects have such serious culminations that the very safety of the home and the nation is involved, for how far can we depend upon individuals whose drug-soaked brains and bodies are liable at any moment to give way under the excessively stimulating or depressing effects of poisons which seep through their veins like a deadly reptile covertly insinuating itself within reach of its prey, ready to strike at the proper moment?

CONSTIPATION—THE GRAVE
–DIGGER OF HUMANITY–

It is not at all singular that in tracing the history of almost all kinds of ailments from insomnia to insanity, that one symptom, chronic constipation, is a common contributory cause to them all. Constipation is an almost universal affliction, but the gravity of it is appreciated by few. It seems to be accepted as a necessary evil and little importance is attached to it. If questioned about the condition of their bowels and the frequency of elimination, many people are forced to give the matter some consideration before replying. Very often they don't know if their bowels moved yesterday or last week, so little heed do they give to this function. The person who values his health and has ordinary common sense about the care of his body knows that a dull, listless, heavy feeling retards his mental as well as physical alertness when daily elimination fails to take place. If this condition is prolonged it causes headache, irritability and nervousness and usually terminates in an acute bilious attack which often forces the sufferer to bed for several days.

Constipation due to foods: Chronic constipation is due primarily and fundamentally to foods. The rough, coarse foods, the unmilled grains, the green vegetables, the skins of fruits, all are conducive to peristalsis. They retain moisture in the gastro-intestinal regions and stimulate the muscular contraction and relaxation of the intestines. This muscular reaction is called peristalsis and without it there can be no intestinal elimination. Since these intestinal constructions are dependent upon the foods eaten, it is only logical to assume that if our foods are demineralized and so highly refined that all the valuable mineral salts are destroyed, then the starchy masses which inflate but do not nourish, that are consumed by millions of people every day, are the direct causes of constipation.

An eminent physician, discussing the relation of *cancer* to food before a convention of medical men some time ago, stated that the dietary of cancer-plagued people was poor in mineral salts, whereas those who were free from cancer were sustained on foods rich in mineral salts. Many causes for cancer have been suggested, among them food. Not the classes of foods, but the quality of all foods after they have undergone the extensive bleaching and refining processes which divest them of their energizing minerals, is responsible for the lowering of the disease-resisting properties of the blood stream which renders the body susceptible to the myriad ills of the present age. Here then, by means of deduction, we find the relationship of constipation to cancer. These demineralized foods are known to be causes of constipation and they are assumed to be causes of cancer. The analogy of constipation and cancer is based upon the loss of mineral salts, cellulose and vita-mines in our cereals and breads. The erroneous assumption, prevalent for many years, was that foods nourish in proportion to their ability to undergo complete absorption. The mistake of this has slowly gained recognition among studious authorities who advocate coarse hard breads, few, if any, cooked cereals and a great deal of bran and whole grains of wheat with fruits and cereals.

Until just within the last few years, bran had become a practically extinct product as far as table use was concerned. Of inestimable value in promoting intestinal health, wheat-bran contains a large proportion of cellulose mineral salts and colloids. The two outer layers of the bran contain more phosphorous, calcium and iron compounds than the other parts of the grain, while the third layer, which is the innermost, contains a special kind of protein wherein the much discussed vita-mines are found. When we buy and consume first-patent flour we do not consume the valuable constituents of the bran for the very obvious reason that the bran or outer coating— husk—of the grain has been done away with in the milling process. Consequently then there is nothing in this highly digestible "white flour" to stimulate the action of the bowels. What we need is more non-absorbable food elements and less of the starchy masses of so-called digestible foods. Because the coarser foods pass through the stomach and intestines and are not absorbed, most people think they should not eat these coarse foods— which include bran, young corn, baked potato skins, fruit skins (peaches, pears, apples, grapes) and the seeds of grapes and raisins, etc. These foods are not intended for digestion and complete absorption. They are to our intestines what gravel is to the fowl; they are the roughage which cleanses the walls of the intestines and is necessary to sweep them free of all accumulations which may have packed up during protracted periods of costiveness.

While the walls of the colons are congested with dried fecal matter it is almost impossible for peristalic action to take place, since the accumulations so completely obscure the small muscular tissues that they are unable to respond to any stimulus they may receive. It will then be readily understood how a constipated condition neglected and allowed to run indefinitely, will rapidly become chronic and lead to serious conditions. In many cases the bowels become so clogged and the tissue so hopelessly diseased that it is necessary to remove large lengths of the intestine to assist the patient's recovery. Close examination of these cases after the removal of segments shows that the mucous lining of the diseased tract was worn completely smooth. The normal, healthy intestines are lined with folds, technically known as rugae, and it is the contraction and relaxation of these muscular folds which move the digested food mass on down through the intestinal tract for ultimate elimination.

Infection of the colons, basically due to chronic constipation, wears these folds down to a thin smooth surface, which, in extreme cases, ulcerates and becomes punctured. The small bowel is less frequently infected than the large bowel as digestion is completed in the first part of the small bowel and the bulk of the contents passes on down into the large bowel where it seems the majority of the functional delays begin. In these cases where persistent infection has existed for years, the colon has been found to have lost its normal appearance and function. The putrefying bowel content has sometimes been proved by means of an X-Ray, to have remained stationary for as long a period as 10 days, disseminating bacteria, toxins and various kinds of poisons through the entire system.

In cases where the infection invades the complete length of the intestinal tract, vaccines and serums have necessarily replaced surgical measures, since it would scarcely be advisable or effective to remove the entire intestinal length. The gravity of these infections of the colon and intestines may be estimated by the report of cases by Dr. Henry A. Cotton, Medical Director of the New Jersey State Hospital, in his book "The Defective Delinquent and Insane"—wherein he states that a large percentage of the insanity cases show gastric intestinal infection or have a history of chronic constipation. A small percentage will show an infection of the lower intestinal tract, which is difficult and complicated to treat. These are the cases which often have developed colonic lesions and require surgical procedure. The diagnosis of such cases, according to Dr. Cotton, will disclose a history of habitual constipation, sometimes alternating with diarrhea and passages of large quantities of mucous. These conditions have been found to have extended over a long period and were existent long before the development of mental symptoms, bilious attacks and abdominal pains thought to be indigestion. That the absorption of the poisons resulting from protracted retention of the bowel content was responsible for development of mental disorders is proved conclusively by the fact that all symptoms of these disorders were effectively banished after treatment, which frequently included surgical procedure. For instance, one case out of many, quoting Dr. Cotton:

A married woman of 44 years—previously healthy, suddenly developed severe attacks of dizziness and vertigo so that it was impossible for her to raise her head from the bed. She had been a victim of constipation since girlhood. The condition had gradually become worse and during the attack of vertigo there was much distention of abdomen and pain. Her teeth were X-rayed and all the upper teeth and the molars and bicuspids of the lower jaw were extracted, but with no apparent benefit. About two months after this she underwent a uterine curettment but the dizziness continued. A special examination of the stomach disclosed colon bacilli and a very low hydrochloric acid content. Autogenous vaccines produced no improvement. A while later the patient's tonsils were removed, after which the dizziness and vertigo ceased for a period of two months, at the end of which time both returned. Two years later radiographic studies of the gastro-intestinal tract revealed an enormously distended descending colon. An extensive resection, or surgical removal of the colon of the left side, was done. The patient's recovery was thoroughly satisfactory, and shortly afterward her headaches, vertigo and dizziness disappeared, and as late as a year afterward she was normal in every way, with no indication of the return of any symptoms.

Another acute case. Psychosis in a young married woman of 28, who had one child. Her attack of maniacal excitement came on very suddenly a few days before she was taken to the hospital. She had badly-infected teeth, and all of them were extracted, and her infected tonsils were removed, with no apparent change in mental symptoms.

She was too excited and uncooperative for radiographic studies of the gastrointestinal tract, but a history of habitual constipation since early childhood directed suspicion toward the colon. This was sustained by the failure of autogenous vaccine and anti-streptococcus and colon bacillus serum to have any appreciable effect. Six months after her admittance to the hospital she was operated upon for colonic infection. Previous to the operation she had been very much excited and refused to keep her clothing on. She had torn up a blanket and draped it about her, Hawaiian style, and claimed she was an Indian chief. She had to be constantly confined to a room with a special nurse in the hope that this would help her. She was good natured, but at times inclined to be violent. Considerable concern was felt about her post-operative care, as it seemed impossible that she would remain quiet and not disturb her bandages.

At the operation, the colon was found to be badly involved, and a large segment was removed. Contrary to expectations, while the patient was restless the first day and night, the next day she seemed quiet and asked that her hands be untied, as they were tied with gauze bandages in anticipation of trouble. Her request was complied with, and from that time on her attitude was normal. Her mental condition cleared up, and in less than a week the change from her previous mental state was remarkable, to say the least. Nine months after the operation she was normal in every respect.

It is safe to say that no clinical symptom is oftener encountered than constipation. It is a symptom of an underlying disorder, and freedom from constipation averts many ills.

Other causes: There are various conditions which are unsuspected contributory causes of constipation.

The gradual absorption of arsenic produces stubborn chronic constipation. Arsenic poisoning is contracted from textiles, tonics, cosmetics, arsenic wafers and ointments for skin diseases. Arsenic is an important constituent of dyes and can be absorbed from the dye in hosiery, coloring matter in wallpaper, carpets, curtains and artificial flowers. Morse reports an infant who was poisoned from the blue lining of its basket.

In 1900 an epidemic in England and Wales claimed 3,000 cases. The origin of the epidemic was traced to beer poisoned with arsenic; the arsenic was used in the sulphuric acid in the manufacture of glucose employed to sweeten the beer. Furs also carry arsenic.

There is constipation due to lead poison. This is prevalent among painters and plumbers and is also brought on through the use of skin whiteners and heavy white face powders. It causes a violent purgation of the bowels, followed by severe chronic constipation, hemorrhoids and other rectal disorders.

Constipation may be a result of strychnine poisoning. The effects of strychnine on the alimentary tract are almost as injurious as lead.

There is also constipation due to mercurial poison, contracted from mercury used as a base for rouge, lotions for the skin, dyes, silver fillings in teeth, blue mass and calomel. Experiments by my friend, Dr. J. Dequer, have shown that positive Wasserman reactions were obtainable in 400 cases of chronic constipation and that of this number, 364 cases returned a negative Wasserman after the constipation had been cured by natural methods— diet, hydrotherapy, spinal treatments, etc. Thus many innocent persons may be branded with the irrevocable stigma of venereal disease and subjected to the very injurious treatment for those diseases.

I am, of course, discussing chronic constipation in these pages—not the temporary condition which may be coexistent with some acute condition of the body which will clear up promptly when the malady of the moment is corrected.

In chronic constipation, evacuation is irregular, infrequent and often very laborious and painful. The excrement may be hard and bullet-like or a dry, hard mass. After extremely difficult passages, attacks of diarrhea are not uncommon. Needless to say, these movements are accompanied with foul-smelling gas and such a strain that extreme discomfort and soreness of the rectum are the natural consequence. In some cases the hemorrhoids become so painful that the patient is confined to his bed for days at a time. Persistent, chronic constipation is usually the primary cause of hemorrhoids except in child birth. The operation for the removal of hemorrhoids is one of the most painful of minor surgery.

Symptoms of constipation: The skin of the chronically-constipated person is usually sallow or pasty and frequently covered with eruptions, due to the absorption of toxins. Bad breath, headache and dark circles under the eyes are reliable symptoms of constipation. Headache seems to be an invariable symptom attendant upon consti-pation. Bilious attacks, with the vomiting of bile, severe headache and faintness are the culmination of prolonged periods of unrelieved constipation. Where the system has absorbed a certain amount of the filth and poisonous accu-mulation of the congested bowels, it revolts and makes a desperate attempt to rid itself of sewerage.

Importance of mastication - Evils of cathartic:. General fatigue, mental depression and the origin of many nervous maladies is more or less due to chronic constipation, although few people are aware of it. As has been previous-ly stated, foods are primarily responsible for a great deal of constipation, but improper mastication is another important contributory cause. If the food is literally dumped into the stomach without being thoroughly masticated and insalivated, it devolves upon the stomach to attempt to do the work which should have been performed by the teeth. *No food* can be absorbed until it has been ground to consistency of cream, after which, by means of an osmosis-like procedure, it is conveyed through the cellular walls of the intestines into the bloodstream. The stomach was never intended to perform the functions assigned to the teeth, and as it is not equipped for more than a limited degree of the milling process, only a very small percentage of gulped food can be reduced to an absorbable consistency, and the remainder is deposited in the bowels, where it packs and arrests the muscular reaction of the intestinal tract. Thus the bowels become overloaded, the individual feels loggy, tired, irritable and headachy, and to relieve this condition he resorts to pills, powders, heart depressors, laxatives, cathartics and aperient waters, all of which have the same effect as dynamite on a clogged flue. Relief is only temporary, however, as the symptom, and not the cause has been treated, and within a few days the conditions are just the same again. These cathartics are one of the worst evils among the list of drugs used for self-medication. The various aperient waters, salts and pills used as laxatives destroy the tonicity of the bowels, dry their natural secretions and lessen the vitality of the organs and superinduce further constipation. The use of cathartics rapidly becomes a habit, and the bowels grow sluggish and inactive and refuse to function voluntarily. Paralysis of the bowels is only a few steps removed from this inertia.

Corrective measures: In many instances mild constipation can be overcome by eating less food. Over-eating crowds the bowels, and by reducing the amount of food the digestive tract is given less work to do, and a simple cure is effected.

Of course, it is better to resort to artificial means once in a great while, to ward off an acute bilious attack, than to deliberately invite a disagreeable illness by allowing the constipated condition to run on without any relief. For this purpose the internal bath, or enema, is far preferable as a means of temporary palliation than the calomel pills, mineral manufactured for the purpose. An enema of warm water retained for several minutes while the patient leans forward in a stooping posture to permit the water to run into the intestines will generally give very beneficial results. It is sometimes advisable to take one waters, salts and vile-tasting concoctions enema to cleanse the lower bowel and clear the way for evacuation of the upper tract. The second enema should be what is known as a high enema. The patient should lie down on the left side, stretch out full length and draw the right knee up as far as possible. Near the lower part of the bowel is an S-like curve called the Sigmoid Flexure, which, when the patient is in the above position, opens in such a way as to permit the injection to flow into the bowels more freely. As much water as can be retained is advisable, to insure thorough cleansing, though often very satisfactory results may be obtained with a pint or quart of water.

An absolutely pure mineral oil is valuable as a lubricant for the intestines, and it will greatly facilitate the bowel action. It must be pure, and possess no purgative properties, but act in the same capacity as any oil which is used to lubricate a clogged, rusty pipe.

These methods are justifiable at times, but any artificial means of stimulation has a tendency to decrease the natural functional activity of the bowels. Even the enema, or internal bath, should not be employed except when it is absolutely necessary, as it may quickly become a habit.

Foods and exercise: The only safe and sure cure for chronic constipation is proper adjustment of the diet and exercise suitably adapted to the individual's needs. Exercises which move and stimulate the abdominal organs and walls will be found valuable in correcting faulty bowel condition. These exercises, in connection with wholesome food, including fresh fruits and vegetables and the drinking of plenty of water, will greatly stimulate the activity of the bowels and restore them to a normal condition. In many cases, if the individual would study his own symptoms he could correct his trouble with very little or no medical attention. An observation of his reactions would soon teach him which foods had a desirably laxative effect, and the diet could be regulated accordingly so that no further difficulty would be experienced. I do not mean to imply that this could be done in all cases, but very frequently, with a little care and some effort, simple cases of constipation can be easily corrected.

Stomach and intestinal disorders due to constipation: It is an absolute fact that ninety per cent of all diseases may be directly traced to some derangement of the stomach or intestines. It is common knowledge that stomach and intestinal complaints are prevalent everywhere, and it is also conceded that all lung troubles, from the simple cold to tuberculosis, are due to lowered vitality, which is often the result of imperfect stomach and intestinal functioning. Dyspepsia and constipation go hand in hand and form the nucleus for a chain of diseases.

Intestinal bacteria: It is a well-established fact that all animals and human beings when first born have perfectly sterile digestive tracts—that is, that there are no bacteria nor germs in them. Prof. Metchnikoff, the eminent scientist, who probably has no superior as a biologist or physiologist, contends that if the colon could be preserved from the invasion of intestinal bacteria, most of the diseases which can be traced to the action of these germs could be prevented. "In addition to this, life could be prolonged," he concludes, "because the greatest cause of old age is the absorption of bacterial poisons in the intestines." The large colon is a veritable breeding place for poisonous bacteria, and unless the putrefactive substances are eliminated, the toxins which generate and are absorbed are a menace to the health and sanity of the individual.

For those who require sensational evidence to convince them, I quote an article by Dr. H. T. Turner, which was published in a pamphlet issued by Tyrrell's Hygienic Institute of New York City:

"In 1880 I lost a patient with inflammation of the bowels, and I requested of the friends the privilege of holding a post-mortem examination, as I was satisfied that there was some foreign substances in or near the Ileo Coecal valve, or in that apparently useless appendage, the Appendicula Vermiformis.

The autopsy developed a quantity of grape seed and popcorn, filling the lower enlarged pouch of the colon and the opening into the appendicula vermiformis. This, from the mortified condition of that part of the colon alone, indicated that my diagnosis was correct. I opened the colon throughout the entire length of five feet and found it filled with fecal matter, encrusted on its walls and into the folds of the colon, in many places dry and hard as slate, and so completely obstructing the passage of the bowels as to throw the patient into violent colic (as his friends stated) sometimes as often as twice a month for years, and that powerful doses of physic were his only relief. They further stated that all the doctors had agreed that it was bilious colic.

I observed that this encrusted matter was evidently of long standing, the result of years of accumulation, and the remote cause—not the immediate cause—of his death. The Sigmoid Flexure, or bend in the colon on the left side, was especially full and distended to fully double its natural size, filling the gut uniformly, with a small hole, the size of one's little finger, through the center, through which the fecal matter passed. In this lower part of the Sigmoid Flexure, just before descending from the rectum, and also in the left-hand upper corner of the colon, as it turns toward the right, was a pocket eaten out of the hardened fecal matter, in which were eggs of worms and quite a quantity of maggots, which had eaten into the sensitive membrane, causing serious inflammation of the colon and the adjacent parts and were the cause of the hemorrhoids, or piles, which I learned were of years' standing. The whole length of the colon was in a state of chronic inflammation, and still this man had no trouble in getting his life insured by one of the best companies in America and was considered a strong and healthy man by his family and neighbors.

As I retired to my room that night, not to sleep, but to meditate upon the revelation contained in that human privy, I naturally went to my eminent medical authorities for causes of disease, to learn if any had given this new revelation and discovery as a cause of disease. I found not even a hint that etiology of any disease described was found in the colon. My memory went back during the years of education and college life and followed along down the after years of study of journals and textbooks of reference to see if, perchance, among all the multiplicity of causes of disease some eminent author had not referred to this human privy whose vault was ever full to overflowing, as the immediate or remote cause of disease, but all were as silent as the grave, so silent that one would suppose that they were ignorant even of the existence of a colon.

Owing to this fact, the prevailing fear of digression from the opinion of authorized authority took possession of me, and for years I practiced my hygienic treatment in silence, only telling a few of my most intimate friends of the conviction of truth that continually revealed itself to me, until my mind and whole being became absorbed with the wonderful truths (although in contradiction to all medical authority) evolving into actual existence from continued experience, until the continued demands of friends and patrons induced me to publish the experience of my life as a result of hygienic and sanitary science, developed in my daily experience.

I have been thus explicit because, out of two hundred and eighty-four cases of autopsy held (they representing nearly all the diseases known to our climate), but twenty-eight colons were found to be free from hardened, adhered matter and in their normal, healthy state, and the two hundred and fifty-six were more or less as described above except, perhaps, the grapes and popcorn. Many of them were distended to in early double their natural size throughout their whole length, with a small hole through the center, and, almost universally, those last cases spoken of had regular evacuations of the bowels each day, many of them (the colons) containing large worms from four to six inches long, producing epilepsy, spinal irritation and extreme nervousness.

My experience, from day to day, develops startling disclosures in the form of worms and the nests of eggs that we daily get from patients, accompanied with blood and pus. As I stood there looking at the colon and reservoir of death, I expressed myself, as my patients do daily, in wonder that anyone can live a week, much less for years, with this cesspool of death and contagion always with him. The absorption of this deadly poison back into the circulation can but cause all the contagious diseases. The recent treatment of hemorrhage of the bowels in typhoid fever has shown it to be caused from maggots, and worms eating into the sensitive membrane and tapping a vein or artery. In fact, my experience during the last ten years has proved, by the rapid recovery of all diseases—especially so-called chronic diseases—that in the colon lies the cause of nearly all ailments. Here is the breeding ground and a fertile soil for disease-breeding germs to be carried from the colon and emptied directly into the lungs, through the portal veins, lacteals and lymphatics by way of the thoracic duct.

It is a well-known fact that physic will not remove this encrusted matter, or even loosen it, but by increased action of the small intestine they are emptied for the time being, giving temporary room for the overloaded stomach and duodenum, and emptying and rinsing out the small passageway through the crusted matter in the colon.

"But why," you ask, "has not this discovery been made before?" There is one main reason. It is that in holding post-mortems this organ was avoided, cut off, if in the way, and thrown into the slop bucket. In the dissecting room the student, taking it for granted that the colon was like the rest of the intestinal canal, cut it off and threw it away, on account of its scent-bag propensities and nastiness. As a result, the profession knows the least about this important organ of any in the human body. Recent investigation has also developed the fact that nearly all cases of tuberculosis have their origin in one or more tubercular ulcers in the colon, located as a sequel of above-described pockets of maggoty worms.

The question is often asked, "Why is this unnatural accumulation in the colon?" The horse or ox promptly obeys the call of nature, and knows no time or place, and are blessed with a clean colon. So are the natives of Africa. But the demands of civilized life insist upon a time and place. Business etiquette, opportunity and a thousand and one excuses stand continually in the way, and nature's call is put off to a more convenient season. The fecal discharge as it is pressed through the Ileo-Coecal valve into the colon is (if natural) of the consistency of paste, and should be but a trifle harder at its final evacuation, but if allowed to remain in the colon longer than three hours it settles into the folds of the colon, and a little remains there, while the remainder becomes hard, and we call it constipation, for its fluid particles have been absorbed back into the circulation. This little, continuing to adhere in the folds, causes, inflammation, and its dryness attracts more accumulation.

Now, this process going on from day to day, from week to week, from year to year, the colon becomes completely lined, losing its nerve elastic power and sensibility. Then the fecal matter passes through the five feet of colon by force of pressure from above like a shoemaker's punch— the first piece cut is the first piece out. That which passed today should have passed one or two weeks ago. Many times, it is small, round balls, hard and apparently molded.

No comment on this highly-lucid article is necessary. It will be a shock to the average mind, which is totally uninformed as to the importance of a clean colon and its bearing upon the entire health. The percentage of normal colons is alarmingly low, twenty-eight out of two hundred and eighty-four cases. This conveys an approximate idea of just how prevalent constipation is.

The permanent cure: The real permanent cure for constipation lies obviously in eternal vigilance as to the condition of the bowels and the discreet consumption of pure food. If the above-described conditions are a result of a cooked dietary, how, then, can we feel protected against the onslaughts of these intestinal terrorists? Since two hundred and fifty-nine out of two hundred and eighty-four cases showed a diseased and chronically-infected colon, it is not unreasonable to assume that there must have been a very definite contributory cause for this condition, which was common to all of these people. Their occupations were necessarily varied, and their habits could not have been identical, but it is a safe conjecture that the food they ate, regardless of their individual station in life, was similar enough in general character to produce about the same results in the system. The foods of the American table, from the lowliest to the most exalted, vary only in the culinary preparation. It matters not whether the foods be served on coarse porcelain or from a gold encrusted china, with the exception of special garnishings and delicate or complex processes of cooking, the mainstays of the table are practically the same—meat, potatoes, vegetables, bread, pastry, coffee or tea. The toxic poisons of the meat, the cooked starch of the potatoes, from which the potassium salts have been carefully boiled and drained down the sink, the demineralized white flour of the bread, the acid-bleached white sugar of the pastry and the irritating stimulants of the beverages, all ultimately produce the same results if persistently adhered to. It may take a little longer where the constitution is strong and the early life has been devoted to vigorous outdoor exercises which have fortified the individual against the inevitable perils of modern civilization. It is just a question of time, however; this slow undermining of health by the insidious, tireless workers which menace humanity, and, like the bogie man of the nursery rhyme, "they will get you if you don't watch out."

Raw foods carry 100% nutrition; the body absorbs all that it requires, and the rest is eliminated as waste. Unlike cooked foods, the excess does not lie in the intestines, an inert mass which putrefies and generates poisonous gases and fluids which are re-absorbed in the bloodstream. The odor of the human excrement, which is ordinarily of the most extreme foulness, will, on a diet of raw food or milk, become odorless, one fact which demonstrates clearly that there is *no* retention of undigested food matter to become stagnant and corrupt.

The author was constipated for thirty years, an affliction which clung tenaciously and refused to yield to any treatment. During the ensuing years of constipation, my bowels moved once in every six or possibly ten days. I resorted to salts, pills, enemas, calomel and various other purgatives which acted only as temporary palliatives.

Hemorrhoids are the direct result of constipation. With the constant strain which accompanies a movement of the bowels during a constipated condition, the lower bowel becomes irritated and inflamed and a form of prolapsis takes place. If the costiveness is only temporary and is soon relieved, the natural elasticity and life of the tissues enables them to draw themselves up into proper position again. However, if constipation becomes chronic and the strain is a regular occurrence, the life of the bowel tissue is destroyed and the prolapsed parts are no longer able to resume their normal position. The intense pain and discomfort resulting from this condition is known only to those who have ever suffered from acute hemorrhoidal afflictions.

I suffered the most excruciating pains from hemorrhoids and lived in constant fear of an operation as the only method of obtaining relief. Being hopelessly constipated and infiltrated with the poisons of the stagnant bowel conditions, chronic appendicitis and intestinal adhesions were only a natural sequence. The pain from the appendix and adhesions was so intense and exhausting that it frequently seemed unendurable. Having to abstain from food because of the pain, I found that I felt a little better and I began to eat less food. I commenced to rely more and more upon the action of water and fruit juices as a food. I drank quantities of water and this, in conjunction with a highly refined mineral oil, sleep, exercise, sunlight and rest was of very material assistance in helping me to rebuild myself.

The most important event at this period was my conception of the idea of Bowel Breathing. I had previously overcome and cured a most stubborn catarrhal condition in my head by first developing my lungs to their full capacity and then learning to drive oxygen into the air passages and cavities of the head. This idea occurred to me—"If I overcame catarrh by forcing the air into the head and oxygenating the passages, tissues and membranes, why can I not overcome constipation by driving the air into the bowels to oxygenate the intestines, stimulate the tissues and facilitate peristalsis?"

Logically it was possible. The more I thought of the idea the more reasonable it seemed and I began to work it out. I labored incessantly for months in attempts to drive the air down into the bowels. It was a new system of breathing and required time to perfect. Eventually, I proved to myself that I could cure constipation with this method of *bowel breathing* which oxygenated the bowels. If this curative process of breathing were then employed in connection with a diet of Raw Food, water, suitable and regular exercise, fresh air, sunlight and sleep, Health would then toe the obvious result.

I proved it all to my own satisfaction. No one had been able to cure the long-standing constipated condition from which I had suffered but I had corrected it by simply burning out the waste poisons with the oxygen which I forced into the bowels.

Putrefied, demineralized, cooked food which stagnates and obstructs the intestines is the cause of constipation. With no purifying oxygen entering the clogged areas what can ensue but a foul and putrid mass of decomposition from which poisonous gases generate and infiltrate the bloodstream.

If people would learn to *breathe* and *breathe* correctly, disease could be not only overcome but actually prevented by complete oxygenation of all parts of the body. In constipation as in many other diseases there is a crying need for treatment of the cause instead of treatment of the symptom.

Bowel breathing will prevent or overcome constipation and its painful companion ill hemorrhoids.

INTESTINAL FLATUS OR GAS

Gas on the stomach and in the bowels is a chronic disorder characteristic of the reaction of *cooked foods*. The organs of the body are thwarted in their functions, displaced, prolapsed and diseased through accumulations of gas which are generated by putrefying foods.

People eat a hearty meal and perhaps immediately, or several hours afterward, are annoyed with eructation of gas. They accept this condition as a matter of course and go on from day to day, not realizing that the constant accumulations of gas are pursuing their course back and forth through the body, are greatly increased with every meal, crowd the organs, distend and dislodge them from their normal positions and cause innumerable diseases and disorders and much misery.

Nervousness, headaches, stagnant circulation, cramps, sluggish mentality, dull perceptions, acute indigestion and numerous aches and pains are due to gaseous formations in the bowels and stomach.

These gases, though they are indifferently regarded, have a very definite power in undermining the health, depleting the nervous system to such an extent that weakness, loss of memory, vertigo, eye troubles, depression, hysteria and even paralysis, where the pressure is *so* intense that a large blood vessel gives way.

Palpitation of the heart is very often caused by intestinal gases. I have seen cases suffering from gas pains to such an extent they were forced *to* go to a hospital for treatment. Every morsel of food or drink which they took into their body was seemingly converted into gas, and the misery which they suffered was intense. Severe contraction of the muscles around the heart and sharp, stubborn pains through the heart areas, which actually shut off the breath for a few seconds, frightened these patients into believing that death was imminent. The natural result of this condition, if neglected, would be a diseased condition of the heart, for the pressure of the gas on the nerves causes surcharging and congestion of the blood vessels and a persistent irritation to the regions afflicted. The great strain on the heart under these circumstances lowers its vitality and changes the heartbeat, making it slower and irregular, or quickened with frequent rapid flutterings and racing throbs. Fainting fits are not uncommon to these conditions, for the sudden congestion due to gas around the heart draws the blood from the brain.

Continuous recurrence of this reaction to gas deprives the scalp of its nourishment, and the hair dies and falls out.

Causes of gas: Any kind of food will produce gas in the stomach and bowels if it is not properly masticated. Cooked foods have a natural predisposition to cause gas, for the reason that they are demineralized and devitalized and the body is unable to absorb or eliminate them perfectly. The accumulations of undigested and fermented food lie in the bowels for days at a time. As time goes on they become hardened and dry and new accumulations are added to the already poisonous mass. Gas is generated in these decomposed masses, as it is in the material when disintegration sets in.

Because they are alive and vital, *raw foods* do not ferment as readily as cooked foods, but again I repeat that ALL FOODS will cause gas unless they are thoroughly masticated. Solid foods should be ground to the consistency of cream and be thoroughly insalivated before swallowed. As has been stated in other pages of this book, the stomach cannot perform the functions of the teeth, and if the food is swallowed in chunks the stomach is absolutely incapable of dissolving that food so that more than a meager percentage of it can be absorbed. The result is that the undigested chunks of food lie inert and heavy, and fermentation shortly begins, followed thereafter by flatulence and discomfort and frequently intense pain. Many people die every year from violent attacks of indigestion. An acute condition is brought on by masses of undigested food in the stomach, and the quantities of gas which generate from it are distributed through the system, paralyzing the nerve centers and congesting the respiratory organs.

All foods contain minerals which are part of their molecular composition. When the foods are crushed with the teeth in the process of mastication, the cells are broken up and the minerals liberated. If the food is not masticated thoroughly but is swallowed in pieces which may have been crushed slightly but not *ground* with the teeth, the fermentation of the undigested food in the stomach results in decomposition and the production of gas. This gas, combined with the previously-accumulated impurities of the intestines and stomach, results in many disorders which vary in character and severity.

The greatest care should be exercised by those living or contemplating living on a diet of raw foods. Because of their highly-nutritious properties and the fact that they are eaten in their natural state, with none of the minerals lost, the raw foods have enormous power and are capable of causing great digestive disturbance unless they are thoroughly ground to a creamy consistency with the teeth. Mastication stimulates the salivary glands and causes them to release their secretions, the mixing of which with the food is essential to perfect digestion and assimilation. The longer food is chewed the more thoroughly it becomes insalivated. Perfect insalivation renders the food assimilable for the stomach and relieves that organ of the over-taxation to which it is otherwise subjected.

Many people eat a hearty meal, so hearty that they feel uncomfortable for a while after eating. Within two or three hours they complain of being hungry in spite of the large meal they ate shortly before. This is due primarily to the deficiency of nutritive value of the foods and secondly to imperfect mastication. The stomach being unable to grind the food to the consistency suitable for assimilation, the nerves are unable to take up all that they require, and while they absorb enough to satisfy them for a short time, they are soon clamoring for more food.

Irritation of the stomach is often misconstrued for hunger. A stomach overloaded or under-nourished becomes tender and sensitive, and the diseased nerves are constantly disturbed.

To avoid gas, which causes disease, discomfort and pain, CHEW YOUR FOOD THOROUGHLY. GRIND it with the teeth and mix it with the saliva. Don't swallow anything until it becomes creamy and smooth and trickles down the throat of its own volition with no conscious act of swallowing on your part. Chew the milk you drink. Also water. Both have more effect in a nutritious way if held in the mouth long enough to stimulate the salivary ducts. The chill   is removed, thus subjecting the stomach to less of a shock, the saliva is blended with the milk or water, whichever it happens to be, and by the time it reaches the stomach it is in a condition which is favorable to perfect assimilation.

If You Wish More Perfect Health:

Avoid cooked foods. They ferment at once, and the fermentation causes gas.

Don't drink liquids with your solid foods. The food is thereby drenched and made soggy, a condition which favors immediate fermentation.

Don't eat bread, cooked potatoes, beans and rice. They contain heavy starches, which also cause fermentation and profuse gas.

If you are annoyed with gas, keep your bowels open, exercise in the fresh air regularly, breathe deeply and completely, massage the abdomen to work the gas down or up.

Fast for a few days to rid your system of the poisonous accumulations. Follow the fast with a diet of fruit juices, alternated with copious use of water. After this treatment let your diet comprise raw foods, the merits of which are expounded in other articles in this book, but remember always, that perfect *assimilation, elimination* and *health* are dependent upon *thorough mastication of all food.*

It is far better to eat often and eat small quantities of food which the stomach can digest than to eat at regular intervals and overload the body. Eat when and because you feel hungry—not because it happens to be breakfast time at 7 A.M., lunch time at 12 P.M. and dinner time at 6 P.M.

If you are suddenly attacked with violent gas pains, drink a glass of water as hot as can be taken. Sip the water in small sips until one glass is consumed. In about five minutes follow with another. Drink the water slowly or more gas will be produced. The hot water alleviates the congestion which produces pain, and causes the gas to move about instead of centralizing in one or two spots.

Beginning in the appendix region, manipulate the abdomen with a rotary movement, pressing the fingers into the flesh deeply enough to move the organs.

Stay in bed under the covers. Lie on the left side with the right knee drawn up as far as possible. This opens the sigmoid flexure, which is a curve of the lower bowel, and permits the gas to be expelled. Apply hot water bottles. As soon as temporary relief is obtained, evacuate the bowels with a high enema. Follow with doses of mineral oil.

SKIN DISORDERS

Pimples, blackhead boils, carbuncles, eczema and all diseases of the skin are simply a manifestation of a system over-crowded with poison which accumulates faster than it can be eliminated.

These various disorders of the skin have their medical classifications and are treated according to the character of the eruption. All skin diseases are the direct result of a poisoned bloodstream. Due *to* cooked, de-mineralized foods, white sugar in candy and pastry, highly seasoned foods, tea, coffee and tobacco, etc., the system becomes overloaded with impurities. The activity of the bowels is diminished and thorough elimination cannot take place.

More poisons are absorbed from the intestinal obstructions and auto-intoxication begins. The poisons and gases thus generated lower the circulation, and the nourishment to certain nerve centers being shut off, those nerves become impinged and inactive. People who suffer with skin eruptions invariably require more oxygen. They do not breathe deeply enough to oxygenize the lungs and purify the *blood.* Their tissues are starved for oxygen and in addition to the poisons they absorb from the clogged bowels, they are also absorbing the poisonous gases which the lungs are unable to throw off.

All of these poisons, plus those which result from a lack of proper bathing of the entire body, have a serious, depleting effect on the bloodstream which feeds the nerve centers.

The function of the nerve centers being impaired the sebaceous glands of the skin are unable to eliminate the accumulations which rise to the surface and the poisons are retained. The resultant irritation and infection of the skin is characterized as a pimple, boil or carbuncle if it is temporary—acne or eczema, etc., if it is more resistive to treatment.

The size and character of the eruptions are dependent upon the amount of poisons retained in the particular centers which influence the locality where the eruption breaks forth.

Cases afflicted with long standing skin diseases have been found, like most insanity cases, to be suffering with a warped spine, with several vertebrae out of position. The impingement of the nerves due to these spinal conditions influence the entire system.

Foods rich in poisons and deficient in nourishment are the original causes of all skin diseases.

It is useless to apply external remedies and take treatments, whether they be massage, electric or any of the numerous methods widely advocated, when the seat of the trouble is inside of the body.

Correct the cause—don't treat the eruptions which are only symptoms.

Clean out the system by a regulated fast where the individual's strength warrants it.

Flush the kidneys with plenty of water, open the bowels with a reliable mineral oil, fill the lungs with oxygen to eliminate the impurities and revivify the tissues.

Take sun baths and air baths frequently. Get as much sleep as possible, rest the body thoroughly and give it a chance to build the strength necessary to eliminate the poisons.

Abstain from all cooked foods after the fast has cleaned the system.

Drink buttermilk. Its action on the skin is most beneficial and it obviates the dangers of intestinal fermentation.

Build the body on fresh raw foods which are vital and carry 100 per cent nutrition.

Eat the crisp green vegetables, the juicy citric fruits, nuts, raisins and whole grains, all of which supply the body with the essential vitamins.

FEET

Scrupulous attention to the feet is a point upon which great emphasis should be laid, as many diseases are promoted by the re-absorption into the body of the poisons which are eliminated through the soles of the feet.

Due to the force of gravitation a vast amount of poison is drained down through the system and eliminated through the skin of the feet.

These poisons accumulate rapidly because the feet are tightly encased in shoes which do not permit any circulation of air. The heat of the shoes induces perspiration of the feet and both hosiery and shoes become saturated with the poisons.

Even with scrupulous care some poison is certain to be re-absorbed into the system. Many people who are fastidious about their personal appearance and give special care to the face, neck and hands, are indifferent to the condition of their feet. They may change their underclothing frequently, but they will wear the same pair of hose for several days.

The re-absorption of the poisons which accumulate in the shoes and stockings, poisons the bloodstream. The resistance of the circulation is lowered, and the vitality of the nerves is depleted.

Unclean feet are often responsible for colds, nervous disorders, aching pains in the back and internal organs, in the legs, ankles and heels.

The absorption of foot poisons affects the sciatic nerve. The effects of these poisons are not limited, and *perverted mental* and *sex* impulses are sometimes the outcome of systemic poison, due to unclean feet. Many skin disorders are due to a system clogged with poison, much of which is absorbed from the feet.

I have found many cases of pyorrhea among people who were so careless about their feet that the odors were quite noticeable when they came to my office for treatment.

People cannot expect to have health even if they try to eat the right foods, treat with doctors, osteopaths and chiropractors and dentists, if they disregard the first precept of health, which is *cleanliness.*

The feet must be kept scrupulously clean if one wants health and a pure bloodstream.

Hose should be changed every day and never worn two days in succession. The poisons which accumulate in one day remain in the stockings and dry over night. When donned the following morning, the warmth of the feet softens the hose again and the pasty accumulations of poison from the previous day's wearing are re-absorbed through the pores of the soles of the feet. Some people have a habit of wearing a pair of hose one day and then laying that pair aside for a day or two, but not washing it. Two or three days later they put on these soiled hose and wear them again. The habit is not a cleanly one and its effects are very injurious.

The same is true of shoes. When one pair is constantly worn, week in and week out, the leather becomes charged with the poisons drained from the feet and these poisons are steadily re-absorbed into the system again.

*Every*one should have at least three pairs of shoes. This will enable him to change his shoes every day and give each pair a thorough airing for two days before resuming the use of them again. The circulation of air through the shoes will purify them to some extent and render them more wholesome for the next wearing.

By giving scrupulous attention to the hose and shoes and intelligent care to the feet, much systemic trouble can be corrected and avoided.

The feet should be washed thoroughly at least once a day and twice, if possible. If they are bathed at night they will need another bath in the morning before the shoes and stockings are put on, as more poisons have been eliminated during the night and should be washed off.

Because the feet sustain the weight of the entire body they deserve as much or more care than the rest of the body, since we are dependent upon them for our activities.

Ask yourself if you are scrupulously clean about your body and give special attention to the care of your feet.

Do you bathe them at least once a day whether you take a tub bath or not?

Do you change your stockings every day?

Do you ventilate your shoes and try to have more than one or two pairs—not for appearance's sake, but from a hygienic standpoint?

Answer these questions conscientiously and see what you find out about yourself. Are you 100 per cent clean?

DETECTING DISEASE BY VIBRATIONS OF THE VOICE AND WALK

In the rebuilding of myself in the past ten years from a weakling to my present condition of health, I have passed through almost all the various stages of disease known to the medical profession—chronic head catarrh, frontal sinus troubles, colds, weak lungs, chronic appendicitis and adhesions, neuritis, rheumatism of the heart and joints, Bright's disease, enlarged heart, partial paralysis of the limbs, from the hips down, and other diseases, many of which have been mentioned in preceding pages.

I watched and studied the conditions that were responsible for the death of my beloved mother and sister and the knowledge thus derived seemed to bring me in closer touch with the natural laws which are governed by a Divine Power.

Through the detailed observation and close scrutiny which my practice necessitated, I was brought to the realization that the great forces of life lay in *vibrations* and that health was dependent upon the rate at which the vibrations passed through the body.

Since *oxygen* is the breath of life, *oxygen* is therefore the greatest and most powerful agency of *vibration* in the body. Without oxygen there can be no *life* in the body, and without life there can be no vibrations. Hence, if the breathing capacity is restricted the vibrations of the body are lowered.

In diagnosing the principal theories of vibrations in myself and patients, I found that ninety-nine cases out of every hundred had a *minimum lung capacity.* The restrictions were frequently of such a character that just enough oxygen penetrated the lungs to enable the individual to live. If the lungs were capable of, a five-inch expansion, then there was probably about one and a quarter to one and one-half of the capacity used. The other capacity was undeveloped. In other words, practically four-fifths of the lungs were atrophying from lack of use. If an arm, leg or foot is not used and exercised, the circulation becomes stagnant in that part, the nourishment is suspended and the part soon withers and becomes useless. So it is with the lungs. If not thoroughly oxygenated they become shrunken and diseased.

In observing my cases closely, I found that the sound of the *voice* was influenced in proportion to the amount of *oxygen* which was taken into the body. Moreover, the physical movements were affected. If the person breathed in a shallow, superficial manner, his walk was slow, his stride short and his general activities lacking in alertness. If he breathed deeply, inhaled and expelled thoroughly, his stride was long and swinging but the walk was fast and all movements of the body rapid and decisive, showing that thorough *oxygenation* of the lungs stimulated the entire *body, mind* and *actions.*

Wherever we find a *keen, alert* mind we will find an individual whose movements are *quick,* actuated by rapidly running impulses. That is a natural sequence. If the mind is working rapidly the body must be in fairly good condition and the stimulus which quickens the mental impulses is also acting upon the physical body.

Neither *mind* nor *body* can be *one hundred per cent efficient* if the *breathing* is insufficient to inflate the lungs to their full capacity. A lack of *oxygen, then,* is primarily responsible for all conditions of the body, except those incurred as a result of accidents.

In the thousands of cases I have personally examined, I have never yet seen a case where *chronic disease* has set in, where the lungs were receiving their full quota of oxygen and, as I have already stated, the bodily vibrations are in equal, proportion to the air taken in the body. Out of thousands of pyorrhea cases I have examined and treated, I have yet to find one which used the lungs to the full capacity and drove the air into the head.

In all cases where the lungs are not being fully used, a dried, stiff and pinched spine will be found, with one to ten vertebrae out of position.

Few people realize that *their voices* are indicators of *disease* and that the condition of the system, aside from those of the organs and passages which immediately affect the voice, have a very direct bearing upon the speaking voice, influencing its pitch, placement, vibrations and quality.

If one is familiar enough with the conditions of the body which affect the voice, it is quite possible to diagnose a case with fair accuracy without seeing the patient, but merely hearing him speak at some length in an adjoining room.

The rather full voice with a slightly dull, pressed quality indicates a reasonably strong nerve tissue and powerful jaws, but somewhat congested head and nasal passages. The possessors of this type of voice do not develop extensive tooth trouble. The *blood* supply to the jaws keeps them well nourished and only superficial mouth troubles are apt to arise.

The thick, foggy voice, placed in the throat, is characteristic of head catarrh, sluggish systemic functions and general internal impurities. These voices are usually so clouded and the air passages so obstructed that strict attention must be paid to understand the speaker. Organic diseases and functional disorders are usually prevalent in cases of this character, for the poisons absorbed from the extreme catarrhal conditions retard the activity of the entire body.

We frequently hear a *thin, squeaky, rasping voice* in a fairly active, well-developed man. This is due to the fact that most of the strength of the system goes to maintain the body and little is left to sustain the voice. There is insufficient *oxygen* to nourish the entire body and the vocal organs and the nerves of the throat become weakened and thin. This condition lowers the resistance of the jaws and head and while the general health may be reasonably sound, the *gums* are subject to heavy congestion and the *teeth* apt to develop serious infections if neglected.

Then there is the thin man (he may be tall or short) with a *deep, powerful voice* which is indicative of strong jaws and well developed vocal cords which receive plenty of nourishment because of the circulatory conditions through the throat and head. His *voice* shows strong resistive qualities, but his *walk* will be slightly stiff and heavy, due to spinal disorders, constipation, liver disturbances. Frequently *scalp diseases* and *loss of hair* are to be noted in these cases. The strength of his voice is due to the unequal distribution of nerve vitality, the majority of which is retained in the throat and vocal organs. The nerve vitality of the general body is thin and weak and unevenly balanced; hence the diseases which characterize the case.

The woman whose voice is loud, high-pitched and of irritating quality, is a victim of nerves, lowered vitality and general systemic ailments. She may have good voice fiber but due to the conditions of the body, the nerves become tense and inflamed. The reaction on the voice causes it to take on a rasping quality and a loud, high pitch. Women thus afflicted will he found to be suffering with organic disturbances, nervous disorders and numerous head troubles, jaw and teeth complications and spinal afflictions.

Breath is *life,* and it is impossible to live and express life all over the body unless all parts of it are *oxygenated.*

Old age, decay and death are the result of insufficient *oxygen, imperfect assimilation* and *incomplete elimination.*

If we fail to get into harmony with the Divine forces which govern the laws of nature and actuate the impulses of our bodies, we cannot hope to correct the conditions which influence our physical and mental capacities.

By seeking the co-ordination of all bodily and mental functions, I succeeded in curing adhesions which I had had in the appendix region for some eighteen years. Through oxygenation of all the tissues, plus perfect elimination and proper organic functioning, I overcame and cured this painful condition. Likewise constipation was corrected. Due to general depleted physical conditions and particular intestinal and colonic infections, my bowels moved on an average of once every six to ten days. *Complete breathing,* which forced the *oxygen* through the bowels exploded the hardened masses of putrefaction, stimulated the tissues and increased the circulation to the intestines, effectively corrected this chronic constipation of thirty years' duration.

By adjusting and correcting the conditions which raise the vibrations of the body, I was able to build a *singing voice* from one of thin, wheezy quality and insignificant volume to a voice of power and strength with an extensive range. Similarly, I cured catarrh and many other odious conditions.

All life and energy is a state of *vibration.*

Vibration is the power of the universe, the Divine Creative force.

There is no *vibration* in a body without *oxygen,* for that body is dead and death does not vibrate.

Only life vibrates.

Oxygen then is the medium of vibration— the great agency through which we receive the forces from without.

Oxygen is *Life, Spirit,* the remedy for all ills.

Your rates of vibration depend upon the *Oxygen* you absorb; therefore your health, your happiness and your efficiency are directly amplified or reduced according to the amount of oxygen which you take into your body.

Wake up your minds! Wake up your bodies!

Determine to live life as it should be lived and as your Creator intended you should live it.

THE CARE OF THE MOUTH AND THE TEETH

Venereal Disease and Its Effect on the Teeth

The medical profession today is taking as active an interest in the diseases of the teeth as the dentists themselves, and a physical diagnosis is incomplete without an examination of the teeth and a confirming X-ray plate. There are still the old-style physicians to be found, however, who are completely satisfied with their own methods of treatment and are confident of their ability to cure all ills and place little credence in the theories of the teeth's relation to health. There is also the antique dentist who has so much faith in himself that he needs no X-ray to assist him in diagnosis. I have treated hundreds of cases, some who had been previously treated for pyorrhea; others who had had difficult bridgework done; still others who had work of an extremely technical nature which was quite impossible to perform accurately and perfectly without the aid of an X-ray, yet all of these patients assured me that they had never been to a dentist who had demanded X-rays and who refused to work without them until they came to me. When operations for appendicitis and the removal of tonsils began to fail as a general cure-all, when the ruthless butcher with only the slightest provocation, left the patients weaker and worse off than before, the victims and prospective victims began to rebel against the general slaughter, and the medical profession was forced to go into a closer study of symptoms and causes, and when a patient had pain, constipation or fits, try to search out the cause instead of treating the symptom by slicing the patient up on the general supposition that his appendix was the cause of it all or that he no longer needed his gall-bladder, or that one kidney would serve just as well as two. People found that very often they felt just as wretched and were just as susceptible to sore throats and colds after the removal of the tonsils as they had been before. From time to time some startling facts came out in the newspapers which ascribed a dangerous malady or sudden death to the poisons absorbed from a badly-abscessed tooth. Physicians and dentists began timid research to observe the effects of the treatment of the mouth upon the general health. If the patient did not respond satisfactorily to everything else that was being done, he was finally advised to see his dentist. Hygiene propaganda of the Health Departments, in newspapers and in public schools, lurid advertisements for mouth washes and tooth pastes, all have had their influence toward awakening the public to the menace of mouth diseases and teaching them that the teeth are as much a part of the body as the arms, legs, eyes and nose and that they should receive scrupulous care, not only because they enhance the personal appearance, but because they are a vital factor in the maintenance of health and vigor. No part of the human body can become more foul and filthy than the mouth if neglected and allowed to run indefinitely without the restorative services of the dentist and the cleansing offices of the toothbrush.

Focal infections are not restricted to the mouth but are apt to attack any part of the body if the vitality is sufficiently lowered to permit of their gaining strength paramount to the countless millions of other micro-organisms which inhabit the bloodstream.

These virulent germs may penetrate to the sinuses, the tonsils, the prostate gland or fallopian tubes and hemorrhoidal tissues, ulcers or malignant sores of any kind.

Decay: The progress of decay is dependent upon the individual's resistance. In some strongly constituted people a decayed area will remain stationary in size for several months, or possibly a year. This is due to the general fiber of the body and the hard structure of the tooth, as well as scrupulous cleanliness of the mouth. Other persons, who

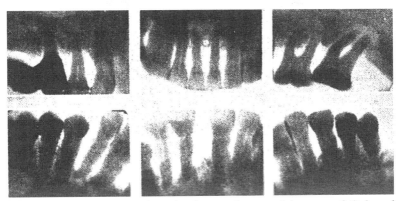

Case 2, advanced Pyorrhea, jawbone destroyed by use of Calomel (Mercury), unmarried girl, about 40 years of age.

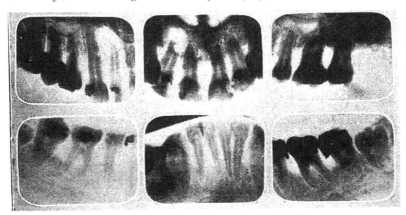

Case 1, advanced Pyorrhea, jawbone destroyed by effects of gonorrhea, unmarried girl, 21 years old.

visit the dentist every three or four months, and keep their mouth exceptionally clean, will have enormous cavities, involving an entire tooth frequently, which will have developed in the intervals between the visits to the dentist. In cases of this kind, the tooth structure is usually of a chalk-like consistency with a soft enamel. At the touch of a bur the tooth crumbles into a fine, dry powder. These same kinds of teeth are often very deceptive, as the external manifestation of decay may be so small as to almost escape notice, whereas, if the tooth is opened into, the entire inside may be undermined with a soft, mushy decay, which has endangered, if not wholly destroyed, the life of the nerve.

Then, there is the individual who never brushes his teeth or sees a dentist, and while his teeth may resemble woolly lambs, he never suffers with a toothache. Teeth of this character are generally set in a strong, well-formed jaw, and the individual having been endowed with a powerful, resistive constitution and probably leading an active life, is able to offset the effects of an unclean mouth for many years. The tooth, having, a smooth, hard enamel, does not decay easily, and consequently the person often escapes toothache for years, but in the meantime he develops pyorrhea, and when the mouth destruction does begin it is usually swift and inevitable.

There are various kinds of tooth structure which are characteristic of certain families, and the teeth may be identical in structure, color and alignment in three or more generations of a family. I have had patients, the grandparents, parents and grandchildren of one family whose teeth were as nearly identical in their distinctive characteristics as teeth can possibly be—the process of decay, reaction to treatment and general endurance averaging about the same. Thus, in building up the strength and resistance of a mouth, there may be not only the individual's peculiarities, but hereditary influences to surmount.

If decay is neglected it eats eventually to the pulp or nerve, which is the vital part of the tooth. A dead or diseased pulp means loss of vitality to that particular tooth, and susceptibility to many physical complications if many devitalized teeth are acquired. Abscessed nerves, improperly treated, are responsible for bone abscesses or granuloma, which may develop years after the original abscess of the tooth was active. These granuloma are a few steps removed from necrosis of the jaw, which is extremely serious and often necessitates the removal of a section of the jaw to insure recovery. Thus we find the development of serious mouth and jaw complications as a result of negligent care of the teeth.

Abscesses: When decay penetrates to the pulp chamber, the nerve, unable to resist the exposure, dies, sometimes very slowly and painlessly, draining the pus and decomposition due to its disintegration, down through the tooth into the jaw. At other times the nerve being extremely inflamed and irritated, throbs and aches violently, spreading the irritation to the immediate area around the tooth and resulting in the swelling of the gums and generation of pus and blood.

This is a highly-active abscess. The procedure in both cases is the treatment and removal of the nerve, thorough cleansing and antisepsis of the root canals and accurate refilling of these canals with material suitable for a nerve substitute. If you have root work to be done consult an oralogist or health dentist.

The slow abscess, the one which works quietly without the individual's knowledge, is commonly known as the blind abscess. Effects of both the active and blind abscesses are easily discernible on X-ray plates by dark, rarefied areas at the apex of the tooth showing where the drainage of pus and poisonous fluids has destroyed the bone structure and weakened the foundation of the tooth.

This diseased area is a fertile field for the generation of the bone abscess or granuloma, the elimination of which requires surgical procedure. The removal of the tooth in no way effects the granuloma, whose poisons continue to seep down through the jaws and into the system long after the extraction of the tooth. Operation for the removal of the granuloma reveals a little pea-shaped clot of blood and pus snugly located in the bone. It is scooped out with a small spoon-shaped instrument, and the jaw heals quickly, and in average cases the patient's general improvement is marked.

Necrosis, which is death to the bone, is the result of a long-standing abscess granuloma, or pyorrhea condition, which has destroyed the life of the bone by the draining of pus and poison down through the membrane and osseous tissues into the bloodstream.

That these conditions of the jaws and mouth have a very material effect on the health is an obvious conclusion. No matter how strong *one* may be physically, the constant absorption of pus and poisonous blood which is being drained into the body is bound to make its inroads on the vitality. The resistance is lowered, the circulation diminished and the bloodstream impoverished, so the impairment of the health is certain.

Pyorrhea: The dentist's great problem of today is the successful treatment of pyorrhea, which is so prevalent that ninety-five per cent of the people are suffering from it in one of its various forms. Failure of the dentists to recognize the early symptoms is responsible for the progress which the disease makes before treatment is begun. The individuals are not always to blame, for while pyorrhea is very often the result of carelessness in mouth hygiene, it is also due to various *local* and *systemic* conditions of which the person concerned is wholly ignorant. When so few of even the reputable dentists are really efficient in the diagnosis and treatment of pyorrhea, it is entirely excusable if the layman takes care of his mouth to the best of his ability and fails to recognize the danger symptoms of gums and membranes.

It is a lamentable fact that some of the worst cases of pyorrhea have developed and advanced to the last stages when the patient was making visits to the same dentist on an average of three or four times a year. I have had cases of this kind, hundreds of them, so I am in *no* way exaggerating. Mouths of beautiful, even teeth have been so ravaged by pyorrhea that the heavy recessions and bone absorption not only ruined the beauty of the mouth but necessitated the extraction of the teeth, which were ready to fall out, but were otherwise sound and untouched by decay, and all this taking place under the very eyes of the dentist. These conditions are not confined to adults but are found in girls and boys just reaching youthful maturity.

Symptoms: The symptoms of pyorrhea vary according to the age and physical composition of the individual and the progress, character and cause of the disease. The local symptoms of pyorrhea are congested, receding gums, the color of which is influenced largely by the cause of the pyorrhea, as for instance, mercurial poison produces a reddish blue, or a bluish purple line around the gums at the necks of the teeth, which is typical of mercurial pyorrhea. In most advanced cases the gums bleed profusely, although frequently one finds a case with a heavy alveolar absorption, with only a moderately congested peridental membrane. Deep pockets around the necks of the teeth, varying in size and depth according to the severity of the case, are characteristic of the disease. Frequently the pocket extends the entire length of the tooth, so that practically no gum or bone tissue supports the tooth, and it is only held in place by the very end or apex of the root, which rests in the bone so loosely that the tooth could be plucked out without the least pain to the patient. Into those pockets an explorer or smooth broach may be dropped from one-half to one and one-half inches, so completely is the bone destroyed.

Quantities of pus can be squeezed from the diseased gums, the consistency and color of the pus depending upon the condition and the cause of the pyorrhea. These are, of course, the local symptoms of advanced cases, although it is not unusual to find a thin, creamy pus in mouths that have not become badly congested nor the bone process heavily destroyed. It is the continual seeping of the poisonous pus down through the jaw which eats away the bone tissue and mucous membrane and destroys the nerve vitality of the body. While a great deal of this pus is

absorbed through the jaws, a large per cent of it is
swallowed with the food and saliva. Upon the necks of
diseased teeth below the gum line are frequently found
dark greenish brown and reddish brown scales, which are
the excess mineral accumulations in the blood, and which
are known as serumal deposits. These are not always
removed by the dentists and cannot be removed by the
toothbrush.

The deposits above the gum line are known as
salivary calculus and are thrown down by the saliva,
indicating that the patient is getting more of certain kind of
minerals than the body can absorb, and it is taking this
means of eliminating the excess. Improper cleansing of the
teeth is a factor in the formation of scales as the particles of
food and mucous left on or between the teeth adhere to the
enamel and gradually harden into a solid mass.

The pus congestion and scales all carry very active
bacteria, and the systemic absorption of these poisons is
bound to have a definite effect upon the body. Frequently
the pus on one tooth alone is sufficient to destroy the
vitality and life of an individual.

There are no cases where a pyorrhea condition is existent on one tooth alone. I have had patients come to consult
me about the condition of one tooth, stating that their dentist had assured them that only that particular tooth had a
pyorrhea infection and that the other teeth were in no way
affected. It is impossible to have rheumatism in a joint of
the finger and not have the rheumatic germ in the bloodstream. The blood which circulates through the finger goes
all through the body. Hence, the bloodstream which feeds
one tooth suppliers all the teeth, and if one tooth has a pyorrhea infection it is only logical that the bloodstream
carries the infection to all the teeth. At all events, if anyone
doubts the logic of this theory (which has been proved so
often it has become a fact), let him have a bacteriological

test made of the secretions around each tooth. He will then be convinced at once that all teeth are affected. If the disease has progressed so far that congestion, pus, bone absorption and looseness are apparent, then you may be quite confident that the X-rays will show the general alveolar absorption which characterizes pyorrhea.

Unless the patient's physical condition is sufficiently strong to resist the depleting action of the pus absorbed from the mouth and jaw, the disease progresses rapidly. This is particularly true in the advanced cases where a few weeks will show an appreciable increase in the rarefied area, so rapidly does the pus destroy the bone.

The local and mechanical causes of pyorrhea are: Malocclusion, under-shod and over-shod jaws common to malformed and irregular teeth; loss of teeth, which throws strain on other teeth and causes them to turn out of position; imperfect fillings, overlapping edges of fillings; ill-fitting crowns and bridgework and plates which do not articulate properly; fixed bridges which cannot be thoroughly cleansed and are therefore unsanitary; tin-can crowns; imperfectly-formed and rough enamel edges at the gum line; then, saw-edged enamel which is imperfectly formed between the teeth and at necks, serrated ridges of enamel; improperly adjusted bite in building mechanical work; the improper brushing of the teeth, failure to remove the foreign matter between the teeth and around the necks, which allows the food particles to accumulate, decompose and irritate the gum tissue.

Poorly-fitting bridges and crowns and artificial plates are another contributory cause of pyorrhea. Single crowns and crowns and bridges which do not cover the entire tooth, but leave a gaping joint between the crown and the gum line, permit food to accumulate. Faulty preparation of teeth for crown and bridgework is a common error. Poorly-fitting crowns and bridges and plates are a source of constant irritation. The subsequent sensitiveness arising from such a condition as this is often the primary cause of pyorrhea in an otherwise healthy mouth.

Partial restorations (artificial plates) which do not fit the teeth properly, rock back and forth and rub on the gums during mastication, injure the gum tissue and wear down the enamel of the teeth. A single ill-fitting clasp on a plate will so inflame the gums as to set up a general imitation over the entire mouth, not to mention the injury to the tooth upon which it rests, which will frequently decay and die.

The gold used in crowns is frequently of an inferior quality, carrying a heavy percentage of copper, which has an injurious effect on the membrane of the mouth and subjects the patient to poison by absorption.

The red rubbers used in plates contain Vermillion coloring matter, sulpur and frequently mercury. Mercury having a strong affinity for the jawbone, is easily absorbed through the tissues of the mouth, and the irritation to the tissues and membranes resulting from the rubber is often responsible for the seemingly unreasonable insistence of a patient that a plate does not fit. Frequently when gold and silver fillings are carelessly put in the teeth they are not properly trimmed down and adapted to the natural contour of the teeth. These overlapping edges being rough and jagged irritate tine gums and tongue and retain the accumulations of food between the teeth. Here, then, is another source of irritation which will produce a case of superficial pyorrhea.

Some individuals, of course, have an idiosyncrasy to the poisons in metals which are used to fill the teeth, as well as drugs which are given in the treatment for diseases. Naturally eccentricities of this kind are prone to produce hyperacidity and susceptibility to complications.

Other local causes of pyorrhea are the picking of the teeth with needles, pins, toothpicks, matches and knife blades. These habits are infectious and are often responsible for serious injury to the gum tissue. Splinters from matches which carry surplus, and slivers from toothpicks irritate and infect the gum tissue when they become wedged in between the teeth or under the gums. Coarse, blunt, unwieldy articles or the sharp points of needles and pins will bruise the tissue and irritate it severely, although the individual may not feel the irritation at the time. The best of toothbrushes will shed its bristles from time to time, and one of these bristles will occasionally lodge between the teeth or wedge itself into the gum around the teeth and set up an acute irritation.

I have also known dentists who advocated the use of charcoal and cuttlefish as a cleanser of the teeth and breath purifier. Charcoal, cuttlefish and pumice are pronounced gum irritants, and their constant use will bring about a chronic inflammation which eventually develops into pyorrhea.

Like cancer, pyorrhea is basically due to a chronic irritation, and to avoid the development of both diseases, it is imperative that we avoid the causes of irritation.

Pyorrhea in an exceedingly bad form is found among the people who do not believe in pyorrhea and think that too frequent prophylaxis by the dentist wears the teeth out. They are content to do their own diagnosing, and unless they have a toothache they don't visit a dentist oftener than once in a year and a half. Through the smug self-satisfaction and stubbornness of patients of this type, many mouths of fine teeth develop severe pyorrhea and are greatly depleted in strength as a consequence when they might, with only normal care, have escaped all trace of the disease.

The congestion and pus which develop in these cases are due to many causes, among which are over-eating, inactivity, lack of sleep, indigestion, poor circulation or overindulgence in sex. The gums may bleed freely but possess a fairly good color and have only a slight irritation or soreness. Due to any one or more of the above-mentioned causes, the cells break down, the fibrin, the corpuscles and the albuminous matter of the blood die and decompose and generate pus.

Due to the ignorance or dishonesty of many dentists who exact large fees for the professed cure of pyorrhea and fail to effect that cure, the average patient thinks he is being robbed or cheated when he is told that he has pyorrhea unless the symptoms are of such a nature that he can recognize them himself from what he has read or heard. This, of course, accounts for the reluctance of many people to believe the dentist when he tells them they have pyorrhea and that it can be cured.

Systemic diseases and conditions are reflected in the mouth, but few dentists recognize or admit the fact. Whether they are loathe to go into the detailed study required for thorough and complete diagnosis or are actually convinced that there is no connecting link between the physical condition and oral disorders, I am at a loss to say, but I do know that the men who take pains to advise their patients of the necessity of health for the maintenance of sound, healthy mouths, are so rare that they are scarcely ever heard of.

Venereal diseases: One of the greatest systemic influences of the present day on the mouth is *venereal disease,* and its effects are as inevitable as death itself. Due to the fact that mercury forms an important part in the treatment of some of these social diseases and because of the affinity of mercury for the jawbone, part of the heavy bone destruction in the cases may be traced to the treatment itself. Once contracted, I am convinced there is no complete cure for these diseases, from a medicinal standpoint, without first thoroughly renovating the body by the proper use of water and oil, oxygenation of the tissues by proper breathing and finally, a proper diet, which is to be found in *Raw Foods.* We have absolute, positive proof in case after case of the complete cure of these diseases by the treatment of *fasting* and a diet of *fruits* and *raw food*. That the virulent germs of these specific diseases continue to thrive in the bloodstream after ordinary treatment, is evidenced not only in the terrific destruction of the jawbone but in the hereditary conditions of the off-spring to whom the effects, but not the active germ itself, are transmitted.

Clinics, hospitals, museums and the streets of our cities and villages are filled with the specimens of blighted humanity that are the hereditary result of venereal diseases.

The medical profession *cures* these specific diseases by suppressing them, but it is universally known that the dormant germ continues to exist in the bloodstream. It does not break out again in active venereal disease if successfully treated, but it manifests itself in other ways, such as loss of hair, diseased jaws and teeth, impaired eyesight, spinal diseases, intestinal adhesions, locomotor ataxia, paresis and insanity and many organic and functional diseases and disorders, the mention of which is limited by space.

There are other processes of deduction by which one may arrive at the same conclusion, namely, this: I have had numerous cases of young people—girls in the early twenties, vigorous young men under thirty or just over thirty, both sexes strong and active, in many instances of athletic accomplishments. The X-rays in these cases have invariably revealed an enormous absorption of the jawbone and great scallops of bone tissue eaten away all around the necks of the teeth across the entire jaw. The closely-checked histories disclosed no hereditary weaknesses, the constitutions being generally strong and the individuals having had practically no illnesses. If the teeth were well formed, as they nearly always were, the jaws powerful and the nerve conditions entirely desirable, the health and youth of the patient would certainly indicate that there must be a great unseen force undermining the natural mouth and jaw resistance.

Heavy pus, extensive recession of gums and bone, with part or all of the teeth so loose that they were ready to fall out, were the characteristic local symptoms of these cases.

With no silver fillings in some cases, and too few in others, to warrant the absorption of sufficient mercury to account for the existing destruction of the jawbone, and no other local irritations of a serious enough character to cause any great damage, what is responsible for this depletion of the mouth and jaw?

The patients when questioned about all other conditions are finally cross-examined as to any indiscretions which resulted in the contraction of venereal diseases. After much protest and denial, they have almost always admitted having had any one of the social diseases one or more times.

One young man of fine physique and splendid constitution had been a star athlete in college. His general physical composition appeared almost perfect, but he had an advanced case of pyorrhea, and the X-ray plates showed an appalling destruction of jawbone. His history was free from disease of the ordinary kind, and the teeth themselves were well formed and aligned. After persistent cross-examination he reluctantly confessed that he had had gonorrhea nine times.

Experiences of this kind are not rare. They have occurred repeatedly. When I had failed to find in the local condition and the case history facts sufficiently strong upon which to base my convictions, I was forced to question the patient on a subject that was certain to be disagreeable and to arouse his animosity. Having arrived this far, however, I was as sure of the truth as I was of my own existence. There is a cause for all conditions, and arriving at the cause is the only way to make a diagnosis and definitely correct the trouble. Before making any assertions as to the source of the trouble in these cases, it was necessary that I be absolutely sure of my ground; otherwise serious complications might result from statements of such a character. Quite naturally an innocent patient would be entirely justified in resenting an inference of this kind and a professional man's standing greatly jeopardized if he indiscriminately implied the existence of such systemic conditions where the patient was absolutely guiltless.

In every instance the patient has eventually admitted the truth. Sometimes it was slow in coming, but when a patient's confidence is secured, he or she will divulge a great deal, even though he is of and extremely secretive nature, once he is convinced that the confidence will not be violated.

This all applies particularly to the cases where the pyorrhea condition has advanced greatly and where the jawbones are badly absorbed; where the general physical history was not sufficiently serious to warrant the severity of the case and where there was little or no mechanical work of a nature to produce the irritation.

Aside from the numerous cases which can be traced directly to the effects of venereal disease, there are countless other cases of pyorrhea which are greatly influenced by this relentless scourge. Often in instances where one would least expect to find it, the contaminating influence is manifested in the mouth, either where the patient is personally innocent but is the victim of heredity or where the disease has been treated and suppressed years before the mouth conditions developed.

The manifestation of *hereditary venereal* disease conditions are: A weakness of the jaws and teeth, making both susceptible to all sorts of complications; tendencies of the teeth to develop unreasonable soreness from the simplest infection; prolonged and continuous aching of all the teeth, alternating from first one part of the mouth to the other, and a general impoverished condition of the tissues of the mouth, congestion through jaws and base of the brain, causing cerebral headaches and various other conditions too numerous to mention.

The ability to diagnose the peculiarities of these cases comes only with long experience and closest observation and study, and unless the dentist has the patience to ferret out all the correlating symptoms and spend time and thought in analyzing the distinctive features of each complicated case which comes to his notice, he will never forge ahead, but will remain a plain "tooth-cobbler" all his life.

About one year ago some professional men informed me that they had been doing extensive experimental work to determine just why the lactic bacteria produced decay in the teeth.

They had ascertained, they said, that it was a lack of potassium permanganate in the secretions of the mouth which accounted for the injurious activity of the lactic bacteria. They stated that it had taken a year's hard study and experiment to arrive at this conclusion. I asked what condition was responsible for the lack of potassium permanganate in the secretions of the mouth. This they were unable to answer.

It has been the author's experience that while the scientific world was busy experimenting to find out what kind of bacteria caused one condition in the mouth and teeth and what kind was responsible for another condition, a great deal of time was being lost, and a great many sound teeth were being extracted without correcting the ailments supposedly due to teeth, when the time might have been more profitably spent in seeking the cause of the disease instead of worrying about the bacteria.

Bacteria of various kinds are with us always. The diphtheritic, tubercular, streptococcus, staphylococcus, pneumococcus, amebic, and influenza germs can be found upon analyzing a drop of sputum from anyone's mouth. These and many other germs are always in the blood-stream, and it is only when the strength and vitality of the individual become greatly lowered and weakened that one class of bacteria gains the ascendancy over all the others and certain diseases develop.

Diseases of the teeth themselves are, with the exception of the local causes which I have previously enumerated, the outcome of a cause which exists in the body. The teeth are the cause only insofar as they become infected as a result of the bodily depletion.

The dental and medical professions at the present time are attributing the following diseases to diseased teeth, abscessed nerves and necrosis of the jaw: Neuritis, rheumatism, melancholia, insanity, colonic-infection, hysteria, irritability, nervous disorders, arthritis, indigestion, dyspepsia, under-nourishment, antrum troubles, catarrh, valvular heart diseases, arterio sclerosis, gall-stones, kidney stones, constipation, tonsil troubles, some skin disease and various others.

Through the experiments of men like Billings, Rosenow and other physiologists and pathologists, it has been proved that focal infection areas at the apices of the teeth or around infected gum margins may very directly cause rheumatism, sciatica, neuralgia and neuritis as well as chronic headache and other nervous affections. They may also act as a contributory, if not the exciting cause, of Bright's disease and diabetes, diseases of the respiratory passages and gastric and duodenal ulcers, anemia and every conceivable variety of disorder which is traceable to disturbed assimilation and lowered resistance.

Dr. Henry A. Cotton, director of the New Jersey State Hospital, has given us conclusive proof of the close relation of diseased teeth to violent insanity, colonic infection and stomach and intestinal disorders. A case of insanity of twelve year's standing was cured in an incredibly short time after the extraction of a diseased molar *when all* other treatment had proved *futile.*

"Hobnailed liver" is another disease which may originate from infected teeth.

Dr. Frank Billings asserts that appendicitis is frequently due to streptococcus bacteria which has been absorbed from a mouth or throat infection.

Dr. Wm. Fitzgerald contends that in his experience with hundreds of cases he has never seen a case of goiter in which there was not originally some infection from a necrotic tooth pulp or from the pus pockets of gums affected by pyorrhea. Cases of epilepsy have also been traced to nerve irritation which was basically due to the presence of infected teeth.

Tooth pastes, powders, mouth-washes and the various *dentifrices* and *drugs* are primarily responsible for a large percentage of the pyorrhea conditions existing today. Most pastes and powders contain powdered pumice stone, cuttlefish and frequently charcoal, which irritate the gum tissue and denude or wear through the enamel surface. The careless brushing of the teeth, accompanied by the use of injurious pastes and powders, will in time affect the strongest gums and teeth. All pastes, powders and mouth-washes contain essential oils and powerful astringents. They are made to be sold and are manufactured by men who know little or nothing of pathological, mouth, tooth and general nerve conditions, and care less so long as their products are in demand. To insure this demand they see that these marketable articles are highly flavored with essences and essential oils which impart a clean feeling to the mouth and sweeten the breath temporarily.

The life of civilization has become so artificial that the diseases which develop as a result, require artificial means for treatment, and naturally enough when the individual whose teeth and gums become sensitive, congested, sore and inflamed from any one or more of many causes, such as neglect, poor mechanical work, plates, irregular teeth, etc., and, last but not least, the eating and over-eating of cooked, *devitalized foods* which poison the bloodstream and wreck the health, he is going to resort to the widely-advertised *pastes, powders,* and *dentifrices* which are reputed to cure all mouth ailments. The relief afforded by these preparations is only temporary, as the cause of the trouble has not been removed. However, a slight relief is experienced, and the clean, refreshed feeling imparted to the gums through the use of the patent dentifrices deceives the patient into believing that he is benefited.

Many of the mouth-washes contain *zinc oxide* and other powerful astringents, which shrink and contract the gums. Great injury is done in cases where a pyorrhea condition has eaten away the bone and formed a pus pocket around the necks of the teeth. The gum tissue around these pockets is loose, and the pus which generates in the bones can be squeezed out with the fingers, and some of it is pressed out by the use of the teeth in mastication. When the strongly astringent mouth-washes and pastes are used they cause the gum tissue to contract tightly about the necks of the teeth; hence where the pus, and any small particles of food which might have lodged in the pockets, could formerly escape because the gum was loose and the pocket open, they now are held in place by the tightly-contracted gum. The pocket being closed, the pus and foreign matter (which decomposes and soon becomes pus) are forced to drain out through the bone. The conditions being greatly aggravated, become worse and worse in the bone and seriously affect the system.

Often to all outward appearances the gums are sound and healthy and manifest no trace of the inward destruction.

The use of these astringent dentifrices in a healthy mouth produces a diseased condition of the gums by pinching the tiny capillaries and stopping the circulation. With the blood supply checked, the gums wither and gradually die and, their impurities being retained, breed disease. I do not mean to condemn all tooth pastes, powders and mouthwashes. Many of them are scientifically blended formulas composed of superior ingredients, but there are ten low-grade, injurious products to one whose merits are worth notice.

Mercury has a strong affinity for the jawbone, and once taken internally or absorbed into the system is difficult to eliminate. *Mercurial pyorrhea* is very frequently due to *calomel,* which is mercury and is given to flush the bowels and stimulate the liver. Contrary to general belief, it is not entirely forced from the system, but part of it remaining, it infiltrates the bloodstream and attacks the jaw. Pyorrhea and heavy destruction of the bone often develops years after the calomel has been taken. One dose may be sufficient to poison a person who has a peculiar idiosyncrasy to calomel. This drug is contained in many pills, powders, aperient waters and tablets given for the liver and bowels. Its effect on the jaws is deadly, and some of the worst cases of pyorrhea I have ever treated were traceable *to* calomel which had been taken by the patient or administered by a physician.

Another form of mercurial poison is contracted through the use of rouges, face powders, skin lotions and skin whiteners, many *of* which contain *mercury, zinc* or *lead* as a base to make them desirably adherent. The drugs are absorbed through the pores of the skin into the bloodstream, and subsequent irritation, congestion and disease of the jaws is the result of the mercury, zinc or lead poisoning.

Lead Poison: One form of lead poison is contracted through the use of sticky, white face powders, lotions and creams which are so saturated with white lead to make them desirably adherent that they will remain on the face and neck for several hours even when the girls and women who use them have gone in swimming.

Heavy powders, lotions and creams having white lead as a base, used on the face, neck, shoulders and arms, produce pimples, rough, broken skin, dry, flaky eczema, boils, coarse-grained skin, large pores, etc. The lead absorbed through the skin and transmitted to the bloodstream, attacks the jaws and produces *pyorrhea* in addition to many other chronic diseases.

QUESTION: How can these forms of pyorrhea caused by mercury and lead poison be cured by just local gum treatments?

ANSWER: They cannot be cured by purely local treatment.

The thorough cure of these conditions necessitates perfect innovation of the system through scientific fasting, restriction of the diet to Raw Foods which carry all the vitamines essential to life and necessary for the complete building of health and resistance in the body.

Over-eating of choked demineralized foods, foods which generate gas, poison the bloodstream, destroy the vitality of the nerves and deaden the sensibilities, is another important contributory cause of pyorrhea. The overloaded body becomes heavy with poisons absorbed from the intestines, where sluggish bowel action has failed to eliminate the waste of the system and putrefied matter is constantly increasing. The result is a general bloating and distension of the tissues, lowered vitality, stagnant circulation of a poisoned bloodstream and a susceptibility to any and all illnesses. Naturally, with the body in this condition, the circulation through the jaws is diminished, the nourishment conveyed to the nerves is insufficient to keep them healthy and the gums and teeth suffering from a lack of nutrition become diseased.

If over-eating is responsible for such ailments as gout, kidney trouble, dropsy, indigestion and dyspepsia, it is also the cause of pyorrhea.

A clean system maintained on a diet of Raw Foods will not develop the conditions which are directly due to the gorging of the cooked, lifeless masses which are designated as food.

Incessant talking, continuous gossiping and the everlasting prattle which characterizes some people is a great factor in breaking down the nervous system, undermining the resistance by draining the reserve energy and generally depleting the nerves. The irritation and congestion through the nerves of the head and jaws which results, brings on diseased conditions in a mouth which is never allowed to rest.

Daily Care of the Teeth

The regular cleaning of the teeth upon arising and after each meal and before retiring requires but a few moments and preserves the teeth and gums and adds years to the life of the patient.

No one thinks of beginning a day without washing his face and hands, even if he is averse to a morning bath. Why, then, will people neglect to wash their mouths and brush their teeth when everything they eat and drink must pass first into the mouth? The very individuals who do this are apt to be extremely fastidious about the cleanliness of their foods (to a point of being finicky), yet they lose sight of the fact that they are contaminating these foods with the filthy accumulations which they carry around in their mouths.

The only requisites for a clean set of healthy teeth are a good, well-made toothbrush, prepared chalk and cold water (not ice-cold nor tepid but just ordinary moderately cold water) and intelligent use of these. The average person scrubs back and forth across the teeth and gums with a sawing motion, which lacerates the gums and gradually destroys the enamel of the teeth. The brush, which need not be an expensive one, but should have a tuft at one end, should be set well on the gums and stroked downward on the upper jaw and upward on the lower jaw. In this manner the bristles sweep not only the teeth themselves, but the spaces between the teeth and remove all particles of food and other foreign matter. This sweeping process need not be made laborious, but if practiced carefully will be found a simple, effective method. The surfaces next the cheeks and tongue as well as the tops of the teeth should be cleaned, and particular attention should be given to the teeth on the back of the jaw to insure thorough cleansing around the necks where food may collect and be retained.

Due to sensitive inflamed and tender gums and teeth, few people are able to use cold water to cleanse the mouth and teeth. After the system has been thoroughly cleaned out, the teeth treated and the mouth condition generally improved, the patient, if he builds himself on the proper foods and lives a life which is conducive to strength and resistance, will be able to accustom his mouth by degrees to a solution of cold water, which will strengthen the gums and keep them firm. A little precipitate of French chalk used from time to time will remove the stains and accumulations from well-kept teeth. There is nothing in the chalk to injure either gums or teeth, and if it fails to clean the teeth then the dentist should be visited at once to ward off possible trouble.

If the gums bleed they are congested. This congestion can often be relieved by squeezing the gum tissues. On the upper grasp the gums between the thumb and index finger, the thumb next the palate, the index finger high on the gum. With a firm pressure squeeze downward over the neck of the tooth. Treat the lower jaw similarly. With the index finger next to the tongue and the thumb next to the cheek, press the gum tissue firmly upward. This opens the tiny capillaries and releases the excess blood, which is usually dark and thick. Squeeze the gums until they stop bleeding. You will not bleed to death. When the blood becomes thin and bright in color, most of the immediate congestion has been relieved.

Everyone should visit the dentist at least every four months, and if the mouth has ever been treated for pyorrhea or had any complications which required special attention, the trips to the dentist should be made oftener than every four months. In consulting the dentist frequently all trouble can be prevented or arrested before it has made serious progress.

Thorough scaling and cleaning of the teeth, which is called prophylaxis, should be performed in a normal mouth every four months, and oftener in a mouth which has been previously diseased. X-rays of the mouth should be made at least once a year to determine the general conditions of the jaw. No dental work should ever be done without X-rays.

Practically all the diseases known to mankind are traceable at some time through the life of the individual to the teeth, which act as a primary cause in producing the trouble. The author funds, however, that these conditions are only symptoms and are not causes.

All troubled, whether they are in the mouth, abdomen or anywhere else, originate in the nerves. Diseases of the hair, teeth, eyes, etc., are the result of the bloodstream's reaction on the nerves. If the bloodstream is pure, the nerves will be strong and there can be no disease with strong, healthy nerves.

In twenty-five years of practice in handling cases of pyorrhea and focal infection and ten years of nerve and body building, my experience has been of such character that it convinced me beyond doubt of the absolute necessity of a pure, clean bloodstream to maintain the health of any and all parts of the body, whether it be the liver, kidneys, stomach, joints, teeth or hair. All are dependent upon the nourishment and stimulation they receive from the blood-stream, and if this great provider is contaminated with venereal disease, the poisons absorbed from cooked, demineralized and improper combinations of foods and the lack of elimination of the same; if the blood-stream is sluggish and impure from a lack of oxygen and complete breathing, if it carries the acids generated by fatigue and loss of sleep, to say nothing of the weakening effects of alcohol, tobacco, tea and coffee and various and sundry diseases suffered at one time or another during life, then most certainly the nerves, teeth, vital organs and, in fact, the general health, are all subjected to degenerative changes which invite serious organic disorders and an abbreviated life.

Here again we find foods as the root of all evil—the foods which are consumed by the civilized races of the world. The barbarian in his savage animal way and due to the lack of equipment with which to ruin his food, unwittingly eats his food in the form which provides him with the greatest strength and endurance. Even though he eats meat and fish, both are generally eaten raw, thereby enabling him to derive the nourishment from the blood of the animal, since it is the blood itself which carries the only nourishment there is in flesh and not the actual flesh fiber, which is only so much waste which the body is forced to eliminate. The *savage eats herbs* and *fruits* and whatever *green products* he fancies which are native to his particular habitat, but he cooks few, if any, of them. If he does cook them they are more apt to be roasted and thus retain their vital elements rather than boiled in quantities of water, which destroy their nutritive properties.

The cook stove is one of the most *damnable* inventions conceived by the human mind, and to its inviting, but treacherous precincts can be traced the source of many diseases.

One great cause of congested teeth, abscessed nerves and extremely sensitive mouths is the alternating hot and cold foods which are served. The shock of hot soups and drinks taken into the mouth incites a rush of blood to the jaws. The subsequent cold shock to the membrane of ice cream and ice water chills the blood and arrests its circulation. The result is a congestion of the gum tissue and the nerves of the teeth.

These continuous shocks of heat and cold are often the immediate cause of the slow death of the nerves of the teeth. The nerve, already congested from the shocks it has received, slowly loses its vitality; the congested fibrin and corpuscles of the blood decompose and break down into pus, and an active abscess is the outcome.

Soft, cooked foods do not require the mastication which is necessary to stimulate the roots of the teeth and increase the circulation of the jaws. Most of the maceration of cooked foods is done with the tongue and only the slight assistance of the teeth. A few snaps of the jaws and the food is swallowed.

Raw Foods necessitate forcible and thorough mastication, and the teeth, which when properly used, move slightly in their sockets, are given regular stimulation and exercise, that strengthens the jaws and extends the life of the tooth. Proper mastication is just as essential to the healthy condition of the mouth as it is to the tranquility of the digestive process.

I have found that foods are fundamentally responsible for most diseases, and, with the exception of venereal diseases, the infections of the bloodstream are primarily the result of a wrong diet.

Demineralized foods, acids produced by sugar in candy and pastry, the heavy, richly-seasoned meats which over-work the liver and eliminating processes, the spices and condiments which over-stimulate the gastric juices, the ex-citing and depressing drugs contained in tea, coffee and tobacco, all take their ultimate toll of the bloodstream. Thus the gradual infection of the bloodstream is brought on by improper foods, and the body, being fed on poison-ous material, is slowly depleted, the nerves lose their elasticity and become thin and susceptible to disease; the resistance of the body being lowered, the functions are ma-terially weakened, and the vitality and strength of the individual are gradually undermined. These conditions, brought on by the foods when aided and abutted by a lack of fresh air, sunshine, exercise, rest and sleep, are simply a combination of forces which lead the victim to an early grave, often after he has led a life of misery and suffering.

Seneca, the Roman philosopher, said, "Man does not die—he kills himself", and this is literally true. The average person digs his grave with his teeth, either from over-eating or with a wrong combination of foods which were improper to begin with.

Pyorrhea is merely a form of *scurvy*—a disease which is produced by the eating of cooked foods. Another disease in the same category is *beri-beri,* and the cure for both these diseases is the consumption of green vegetables, so it would seem only logical that the plentiful eating of green vegetables would serve to immunize against pyorrhea.

I have observed that practically all cases of pyorrhea eat but few citric fruits and very few green vegetables. Those who do include a large supply of fruits and veg-etables in their diet do not manifest pyorrhea in its extreme forms. They may develop light, superficial cases which are primarily due to local disorders, but these people seldom, if ever, suffer the heavy alveolar absorption and general oral depletion which others are wont to do who live on a diet comprised largely of cooked foods.

In my experience with all cases of pyorrhea I have found that the individuals were addicted to the eating of heavy cooked foods with only an occasional bit of celery, lettuce or onions, which were so rarely eaten that they were insufficient to offset the serious disadvantages incurred through the consistent consumption of cooked foods.

The Government reports issued by the U. S. Bureau of Chemistry, Department of Agriculture, defines the three vitamins which are found in all foods as—the water soluble A, the fat soluble B and the anti-scorbutic. The report goes on to state that the best source of the vitamins is in the leafy parts of the green vegetables. This report shows that a quantity of all three vitamins are found in practically all foods but the anti-scorbutic vitamin is found in more abundant quantities in green vegetables—lettuce, tomatoes, oranges, peas, beans, lemons, nuts and cereal.

The report further states that the *drying of these vegetables* and fruits destroys a portion of the vitamins and only a part of them is left. Now, if the drying process, which is widely regarded as scientific and healthful, since dried or dehydrated vegetables and fruits are extensively advocated for their great nutritive merit; if this drying destroys a part of the vitamins, what happens to the vitamins when the vegetables are immersed in water and cooked until they are a shapeless, watery mass?

Is it reasonable to believe that any of the vitamins, at least any part which is sufficient to have a pronounced beneficial effect can remain in the foods after the firing process? The answer stares us all in the face at every turn we take. The people on the streets, the crowds in shops, theatres, and churches, the workers in offices, the sufferers in hospitals and institutions for the blind, crippled and insane, all are living evidences of the appalling lack of vital force in cooked foods and the effects of demineralized products.

Very little is known of the exact nature of the organic elements contained in vitamins, but science has furnished us with convincing proof that these mysterious elements are most essential to the health of every part of our bodies. In this case, then, there must be in the different vitamins, sufficient material to meet the requisites for the teeth, hair, skin, et cetera. If we destroy the vitamins by cooking the foods, how are the various parts of the body to receive the proper nourishment? A normally strong organ may manage to derive some benefit from what small quantity of vitamins may survive the cooking process, but it is certain that this quantity will be insufficient to meet the requirements of all parts of the body; consequently the result will be that those which are starved and deprived of their greatest needs will eventually fail to maintain their standard of health and fulfill their functions. The teeth will decay, the hair fall or turn white, the skin wither and dry and the abdominal organs sag and become diseased.

In order that the child be properly nourished and be fully developed, it is of the utmost importance that the prospective mother eat the foods which contain the highest percentage of life-giving elements, as she herself must absorb some nourishment as well as supply the child's food. Do you think she can nourish herself and her baby solely on cooked foods? That these prospective mothers do not obtain nourishment sufficient for themselves and their babies is evident by the loss of hair and depletion of the teeth which follows maternity. If the bloodstream were supplied with all the elements necessary to the life of the hair and teeth, the destruction of the cells would not take place and the hair and teeth would retain their health and vigor.

In some cases of growing children the condition of whose teeth indicated a deficiency of calcium in the system, I have advocated pulverized egg shells mixed with the food or taken regularly as any medicine might be. If this treatment is continued for several months or a year, where a lack of calcium is indicated, the teeth will be greatly improved in structure and strength.

My success with the treatment of pyorrhea and regeneration of the jaw bone and nerve and body rebuilding has been chiefly due to correct diagnosis to begin with and the co-operation of the patient during and after treatment in adhering closely to my instructions regarding foods, rest, exercise and care of the teeth and the general routine of the daily life.

The surgical treatment of the teeth includes the removal of the scales, the extraction of the worst abscessed teeth if the patient's condition is so serious that every precaution need be exercised for the sake of his health, and the thorough treatment of all other less menacing abscesses, the curetting and sterilizing of all pus pockets, the elimination of pus and the proper attention to all teeth with cavities and the construction of such removable restorations as each case requires.

The patient, immediately after diagnosis and upon the beginning of treatment, is instructed in the matter of Raw Foods, rest, sleep, exercise, fresh air and mental equilibrium, to say nothing of the advice on mouth hygiene and the scrupulous care of the teeth.

Quantities of drinking water are prescribed, and the patient is required to take the water on a regular schedule as though he were taking medicine, for 99% of all pyorrhea and nerve-depleted cases are water-starved and have a dried, leathery skin, poor color and bad circulation. Water is a food, and if properly taken is a valuable aid in flushing the poisons from the system through the kidneys and pores of the skin, oxygenating the tissues, changing the color and heightening the circulation.

The effects, if all instructions are carefully followed out, are to be noticed almost at once, and only by impressing the patient with the seriousness of the case and necessity of the changes, can one hope to secure the full co-operation of the patient.

Some patients will regard the matter seriously for a time and, due to their greatly-improved condition, will slip back into their old habits, thus inducing the return of conditions which provoked their troubles with teeth and jaws, as well as other parts of the body. Other patients, more thoughtful of their health, will live in a manner that is conducive to health of mind and body, and, the original source of their pyorrhea trouble having been removed; they enjoy sound health and freedom from disease as long as they consistently apply their knowledge of how to care for their bodies.

Again I repeat that diseases of the teeth are only responsible for diseases of the body in-so-far as they react conversely in proportion to their own infections which are a result of the lowering of the bodily forces and resistance.

If the teeth are to be kept strong and free from infection, then, aside from the oral hygiene, the general health must be safeguarded. To insure a pure bloodstream and vigorous health, the foods, which build both, must carry 100% nutrition. Devitalized, highly-refined and commercially-processed foods do not carry the nutrition sufficient to build a healthy bloodstream and a robust body.

Raw foods in the state which nature grows them, the foods which sustain the most powerful animals, are the foods which will also sustain mankind and develop him to his highest efficiency.

The ox, which lives on grass and grain, has more power and endurance than the lion, which feeds on flesh. Animals are never diseased except when they are forced to live in civilization. Left to themselves, they seek and find the foods which are good and wholesome and shun what is injurious, but man, by his excesses in food and drink and other manifold dissipations, becomes diseased and ailing and lives out only one-fourth of his allotted time.

BREATHING

All Disease Is Due to a Lack of Complete Oxygenation

"Theoretically, we all desire to live long and be happy. In actuality, we live miserably and briefly."

"The staff of life is breath not bread."
—Estes.

No man, woman or child can be said to be living unless he breathes deeply and correctly —he is merely existing—he is not radiating vitality and energy—he cannot, since he is getting only a minor percentage of the great factor necessary to create these forces. *Oxygen* is the marvelous *builder* and *purifier* which envelops us constantly but which we either overlook completely or give small heed to. To benefit by this great element we have only to learn the simple secrets to correct breathing and train ourselves to absorb the powers of the oxygen forces around us.

Rhythmic breathing: The people of the far East, the Orientals, have for centuries practiced the art of deep breathing, have known its wonderful physical benefits and experienced its spiritual and psychic effects to such an extent that their mysterious occult rituals are entered upon through a preliminary phase of deep breathing which assists them in vibrating into the super-conscious state. Brahman and Buddha gave to their followers instructions in deep breathing, and the Hindu Yogis have used scientific breathing for generations. They designate this scientific breathing as rhythmic breathing. The rhythm of the pulse is ascertained and they practice until the rhythm of the breath corresponds to that of the heartbeat. This rhythmical breathing brings the individual into the harmonious vibrations with nature and the inherent powers which have lain dormant within him are gradually unfolded.

The controlled breath as taught and practiced by myself and thousands of followers cures and prevents disease in the breather himself and banishes fear, worry and the baser emotions. It lends poise and a steady calm, which is conducive to self-confidence and steadfastness of purpose.

The first thing a baby does upon birth is breathe. After it has learned to breathe it promptly sinks into a deep slumber. About the second or third day it begins to eat. All the time the child is sleeping it is breathing deeply. When it awakens and eats it goes back to sleep again. Thus for several months its life is a continuous chain—breathing, sleeping, eating—building, building, building.

During early infancy the child breathes properly. The air is carried down into the lungs, inflating them fully, but as the child develops, it seems to become imbued with the lackadaisical spirit of its *elders*, and gradually the breathing becomes more and more shallow.

Few people naturally breathe deeply. It is a habit which is acquired only by persistent cultivation.

Air is food, a life-sustaining element the same as water, and while we can *live* for weeks without food, several months without water, we cannot live ten minutes without air.

Oxygen a purifier: No lasting, perfect health can be attained without deep breathing. It is absolutely essential to body-building. There is *no* better builder or purifier than oxygen. Let us review its part in purifying the blood. The blood, driven by the heart through the arteries, is fresh, vivid in color and rich in quality; from the arteries it is sent into the tiny capillaries all over the body. Coursing through the arteries and network of capillaries, this rich blood brings new life and nourishment to the body, constantly rebuilding and strengthening it. On the return route, the blood passes into the veins, picking up the waste of the system and no longer carrying the life-giving qualities. It has now lost its full, rich color, is a dull bluish hue and thinner in consistency than before. Now the course directs the blood to the right auricle of the heart, which contracts after it is filled and forces the bloodstream into the right ventricle, which in its turn passes it on to the lungs. After reaching the lungs the blood is distributed by the tiny blood vessels to all the air cells of the lungs. Now, when a breath of air is inhaled, the oxygen is brought into direct contact with the impure blood, which has just left the veins and been conducted Ito the lungs. The hundreds of small blood, vessels of the lungs have very thin walls, which are thick enough to hold the blood but thin enough to permit the oxygen to penetrate them. Thus the oxygen comes in contact with the blood, a form of combustion takes place;, and the oxygen is absorbed into the blood, which in turn throws off a carbonic acid gas generated from the waste products and poisonous matter which has been collected by the blood as it traversed its course over the entire body. Now, the blood is purified after going into the left auricle, being forced into the left ventricle and out and is ready to repeat its journey through the arteries and back again. Since it is the oxygen which purifies the blood by entering the bloodstream, causing the explosion which forces out the poisonous gas, it is obvious that the blood cannot be thoroughly' clarified unless sufficient oxygen is carried into the lungs to perfectly inflate them and reach every part of the lung tissue. How many people breathe deeply enough to permit this complete inflation? Due to carelessness, ignorance, tight clothing or general indifferences nine out of ten people seldom draw a breath below the collar-bone. Observe those about you in the car or theatre. How many chests do you see rising, falling, with the even rhythm of the well-regulated deep breath? Very few.

Unless the breath is deep enough to carry sufficient oxygen to purify the bloodstream, the body is being fed on poisonous material, and we are re-absorbing the impurities which accumulate as the blood pursues its way over and over again. As it completes its circuit three times every minute, one may estimate the rapidity with which these poisons accumulate. It is not a pleasant thought to entertain —feeding the body on rejected filth of the system! You would shudder at the revolting suggestion of eating unclean food, yet you allow your poor, helpless nerves to feed on thin, poisonous blood just because of negligence on your part to exert a little effort and purify that blood with more oxygen.

One-third of all the poison generated in the body is excreted through the lungs, the balance through the bowels, skin and kidneys. Shallow breathing throws a back-wash of poisons upon the other organs of elimination, which become exhausted and clogged from overwork, and finally function but slightly.

Investigation discloses that less than ten per cent of the people breathe correctly.

Disease attacks only the unused lungs, and the deep breather will not be found susceptible to every slight ailment.

Deep breathing for singers and speakers. Aside from a standpoint of health, correct breathing is of inestimable value in the development of orators, singers, athletes and actors. It strengthens the muscles of the throat, chest, diaphragm and abdomen and gives the speaker or singer perfect muscular control, which produces a clear, resonant voice that can be used for hours without fatigue and hoarseness.

Classifications of Breathing I have never yet found any case afflicted with a disease, no matter of what type or character, where true lungs were used to the full capacity and where there was complete breathing and oxygenation. If there were complete breathing and oxygenation, then there could be no disease, for oxygen is the purifier which turns out the waste of the body and obviates disease.

According to the system which I have worked out, breathing may be classified as follows, and explained according to the purpose and function of each class:

Abdominal breathing stimulates the abdominal organs, vibrates the gall bladder, diminishes the dangers of congested and diseased kidneys, bladder, intestinal ulcers, etc. It stimulates and strengthens the muscles of the abdomen, making them firm and tight instead of soft and flab.

Intercostal breathing exercises the heart, stimulates the lower lung areas and develops the diaphragmatic muscles.

Thoracic breathing stimulates the upper lungs, exercises and strengthens the muscles of the center of the trunk, the chest, the busts, the arms, shoulders and back, fills out scrawny necks, shoulders and chest to their proper proportions.

Throat breathing: The air being driven in, the throat may be manipulated with the hands while it is retained. This vibrates the bones of the throat and stimulates all the tissues. It is a means of overcoming throat and tonsil trouble, bronchial infections, diseases of the thyroid gland, as for instance, goiter; also it will keep the throat in such a healthy condition that tendencies to tubercular glands may be obviated.

Face breathing. The breath is held and driven into the tissues of the face, heightening the circulation to the face tissues and inflating them. This stimulation increases the functions and color of the skin, tightens the face muscles, drives out the impurities of the pores, fills out the hollows caused by sagging flesh and restores the face to its youthful contour and freshness. Wherever you see a sallow, sagging face you may know that the body is slowly dying from lack of oxygenation.

Head breathing drives the air through the ethmoid and sphenoid bones, the frontal sinus cavities and the antrum of Highmore, wherein so many dangerous infections of the head cavities have their source. These cavities are all aerated. The air is brought forward and higher than in face breathing and the resultant stimulation cures and prevents cold, catarrh, adenoids, polypus, tonsil trouble, weak eyesight, poor hearing and mal-formed jaws. If parents realized the importance of instructing their children in the necessity of head breathing, there would be fewer under-shot and projecting jaws, mal-posed teeth and generally imperfect oral developments.

Brain breathing is different from head breathing. Head breathing stimulates the frontal cavities and orifices of the head while brain breathing stimulates the large nerve centers of the brain in the top of the head. Brain breathing burns out the waste accumulations thrown off by the mental activities, it affords stimulus for new impulses, quickens the brain, increases the circulation to the scalp and prolongs the life of the hair cells. *Bald headed* people receive no oxygen in the tops of their heads. Their blood pressure is either abnormal or subnormal, a condition which is responsible for malnutrition and loss of pigmentation in their hair. Thorough oxygenation of the brain revivifies the hair cells in the scalp, restores pigmentation to the scalp and increases the growth of the hair.

Bowel breathing exercises the abdominal organs but its primary function is to stimulate peristalsis by increasing the activity of the intestines, The muscles of the groin are exercised and the glands which supply strength to the generative organs are invigorated by regular bowel breathing. Constipation, gas, colonic infection, intestinal catarrh and adhesions may all be cured or prevented by bowel breathing. Anyone who learns bowel breathing need not fear operations for appendicitis, ovarian and gland conditions, as these menacing conditions do not develop where the intestines and bowels are thoroughly oxygenated. The stubbornness cases of constipation yield to the effects of bowel breathing and the system is purified by means of perfect elimination due to this curative breathing process.

Complete breathing. And the final link which completes this cycle of breathing is the complete breath, the unification of all the breaths. After one has learned abdominal, intercostal, thoracic, throat, face, head, brain and bowel breathing, and the science of oxygenating each of these parts, separately, the next step is to practice this system of breathing until one breath oxygenates all the areas simultaneously. This is called the *complete and tissue breathing.*

The object of the complete breath is to distribute the oxygen not only to the *organs* but to the *tissues* of the body thereby stimulating organic functions, tithe nerve centers, the skin, the hair and all parts of the body. After studious practice the *complete and tissue breathing* becomes automatic and with a single effort poisons of the body are burned out and disease is eliminated, or the chances for its contraction are reduced to a minimum.

This all inclusive breathing employed in conjunction with 100% foods, regular exercise and sleep is the direct pathway to Health. The individual who forms these healthful habits is taking medicine every minute of the 24 hours each day and need have no fear of hospitals or graveyards.

This system of curative breathing I have worked out and perfected as a result of the study and cure of my own diseases. I am the originator of *Complete and Tissue Breathing* and I have taught it all over the country, demonstrating to my classes the manner in which oxygen can be driven from the tips of the fingers and the top of the head down to the feet. The tissues off the face, the myriad little veins and muscles in the neck, shoulders, arms, back, legs, knees, ankles and feet can be distended with oxygenated blood by means of the complete breath.

The *complete* and *tissue* breath oxygenates the entire body inside and out.

There can be no disease with complete oxygenation, the body may starve for food, the cells will consume each other and eventually burn up but if complete oxygenation is taking place, there will be no disease. Oxygen is the Spirit-force and where there is oxygen, there is Life, not Death.

The average man breathes abdominally, lightly. The average woman breathes according to the clothing she has on. Her breathing may vary and include from time to time a slight abdominal breath, a pinched intercostal breath and a high thoracic breath.

The use of tobacco in cigars, cigarettes and pipes inhibits complete oxygenation and interferes most seriously with the functions of the respiratory system. Men have, through long habit, become somewhat accustomed to tobacco poison, although they in no way escape its disastrous effects upon the system, but due to the natural strength of their sex and their more exposed lives, they are able to offset its results for a protracted period. The contemptible and increasingly prevalent fad of smoking among women is undermining the health, mentality and refinement of the womanhood of the world. The delicate mechanism of a woman's body was never created to withstand the use of a coarse-grained and insidious drug like tobacco. Neither can it be said that man's was. Smoking is offensive in a man—in a woman it is odious and disgusting. It constricts the lungs, arrests the breathing and induces hundreds of ills, the most deadly of which is *tuberculosis, a disease which never develops in completely oxygenated lungs* Tobacco first stimulates and then depresses; it warps the brain and stunts the development of mind and body, destroys the balance and lowers the vitality. Because of its restricting action upon the organs of respiration alone, it should be avoided like a plague.

Correct breathing cures many ills. The habitual practice of deep breathing greatly obviates the dangers of nose and throat troubles, such as polypus, adenoids, tonsillitis and nasal catarrh. One of the causes of head catarrh is improper breathing. Through lack of inflation of the tissues by the deep, full breath through the air passages, the tissues congest, the air channels are reduced in size, and the breathing becomes labored and audible. Mucous and the natural secretions accumulate and cause the breath to become heavy and offensive with the poisonous odors emanating from the congested areas. Polypus and oseous growths form, necessitating operations which are only too frequently unsuccessful and by no means correct the trouble.

A great deal of annoyance, pain and embarrassment might be avoided through the early instruction in deep breathing.

People who practice deep breathing in the correct way are the possessors of strong lungs, elastic muscles, clear eyes and well-balanced brains. They are beautiful, powerful and successful.

Learn to breathe properly!

Join one of Dr. Estes Back to Nature courses on Brain Breathing and Dynamic Breath Controls. Read all available literature; study special books on the subject; thoroughly acquaint yourself with this most important function of life.

When you have learned how to breathe, *apply* the knowledge and observe your steady improvement.

SLEEP—NATURE'S BLESSED
ANTIDOTE FOR PAIN AND SORROW

It is a common experience to meet people who are, to the best of their knowledge eating the proper food, exercising and caring for themselves in every possible way, yet they complain of feeling tired and they show traces of fatigue; drawn, haggard lines mar the smoothness of their faces, a lagging step, and every movement of the body indicates the greatest effort. These are the signs of a hidden cause which is undermining their stability.

Detailed examinations disclose no organic disorders and to all appearances their health is all that it should be. In instances of this kind SLEEP is the minus quantity—the curative agent needed to forge the final link in the chain of perfect co-ordination.

Effects of loss of sleep: Sleep is the restorative which we all require. Few people ever take an over dose. Tired, fagged nerves shrieking for sleep, will be appeased with no substitutes. The strength and nourishment which accrues to the nerves with nine and ten hours of regular, undisturbed sleep every night will cause the muscles of the face and body to tighten, lift sagging cheeks and erase deepening lines around mouth and eyes. After continued loss of sleep, the nerves lose their vitality, become thin and dried, the eyes become smaller, less vivid in color and the lines of the face and body droop. A plump round face will take on a hollow drawn look, due to the fatigue poisons which are being generated and absorbed and the skin will become sallow, anaemic and leathery.

A few weeks of regular unbroken rest will produce a remarkable change in most people who are tired and over-worked—mentally or physically. Many people say they work all day and desire change and relaxation at night instead of so much sleep. A reasonable amount of relaxation is advisable, but a practical view of these problems must be taken. Unless you are thoroughly rested, how can you thoroughly enjoy your diversions? Haven't you frequently sought relaxation in the form of amusement—movies, theatres, etc., and found yourself too exhausted to derive much pleasure from the performance?

No matter how strong the physical body, the brain will not function as clearly if there be a persistent habit of keeping late hours. True, we may form the habit of going to bed after midnight, "get by" with it for many years, attend to our duties and insist that we feel perfectly all right. But the breaking point will come eventually. It is inevitable.

Sleep before midnight. Those who are familiar with the laws of the universe know that we derive our life forces from the world without—that we are merely mediums through which the various life currents flow. The power we obtain is in the ratio of our physical ability to receive. In other words, any medium must be in receptive condition. If we set up a radio outfit, our messages are much more satisfactory if the delicately constructed mechanism is carefully erected and connected than if it is carelessly set up, with little knowledge of the intricate details of the outfit.

The hours of sleep before midnight are those which count the most. The elemental and astronomical changes are taking place, and from midnight until about 3 o'clock (the zero hour) all vegetable and animal life is at its lowest ebb. The night is waning and a new day is beginning; all life which has lain dormant during the night begins to stir and prepare for the coming day. The crisis in illness often culminates at this hour and a change either for better or worse is noted.

Before midnight the human body is absorbing and drawing to itself the life-sustaining elements of the universe and regeneration is taking place. Hence, if we wait till the elemental changes are transpiring, the forces which we attract to ourselves are diminished in power and we do not derive the strength and sustenance required to replenish the bodily needs.

You may retire at 2 or 3 o'clock in the morning and sleep soundly until noon the following day but you will not feel as refreshed and vigorous as you would had you retired at 8 or 9 in the evening and arisen at 5 the following morning. The people who reach the century mark, leading full active lives and possessing all their faculties, despite their mature years, are invariably advocates of the old adage—"Early to bed and early to rise." Their lives are eloquent testimonies of the value of this precept. With few exceptions, most animals retire early and as evening descends in the wilderness, where no man-made regulations change night into day, the hush which descends with twilight, indicates that all nature goes into retirement for the duration of the darkened hours.

Sleep is a most important agent in the treatment of nervous disorders and although it is frequently difficult to induce regular unbroken slumber, it can be accomplished through the administration of quieting warm baths and soothing drinks before retiring. The sleeping quarters should be thoroughly ventilated at all times and the windows thrown wide open to permit the circulation of all possible fresh air for the sleeper.

Loss of sleep one cause of acidosis. The persistent loss of sleep causes the formation of an acid, the constant absorption of which dries the natural secretions of the joints, particularly the vertebrae, and is responsible for such diseases as neuritis, rheumatism and arthritis deformans. These heavy acids in the circulatory stream also tighten the muscles, thin the nerves and cause impingement of the nerves.

Premature old age, irritability, neurosis, pyorrhea, gum and tooth trouble, tight muscles, stiff spine, taut muscles, dyspepsia, indigestion and general fatigue, while they may not always be directly due to, are frequently super-induced by a long continued loss of sleep. With a sleep-starved body it is impossible to correct such disorders as indigestion, dyspepsia and functional ailments. Sagging muscles, flabby breasts and hips are other manifestations of improperly rested nerves. It is impossible to grow the *hair* again when it has once been lost unless the body is sufficiently nourished with *sleep,* so that cell life is regenerated in the hair follicle.

Sleep a builder of will-power. Sleep is more important than food in cases of extreme exhaustion and depletion. Patients whose vitality has become so lowered are not able to begin even preliminary exercises of deep breathing and exercise. They are so fatigued that they have not the moral power to breathe or eat properly. They are practically dead and the only recourse for them, if they hope to build, is to sleep and rest until the nerves and tissues are able to recuperate.

People who continue to go along the same old ruts of life, even when they know and believe that the more advanced methods are those by which they would receive the greatest benefit, simply have not the will power to put their convictions into execution. They are so undernourished as a result of their demineral-ized foods and so depleted from loss of sleep and lack of rest that no matter how willing they may be to change their mode of living, they have not the moral stamina to begin and they are always planning to do things tomorrow. This procrastination continues for so long that finally tomorrow never comes.

If you would have dynamic energy, force and indomitable will power, see that your body is rested amply and given opportunity for restoration by at least eight hours' sleep each night—and more, if it is subject to any unusual strain.

Sleeping alone: Another important fact of which a great many people are ignorant and to which others give little credence if they are cognizant of it, is that everyone should sleep alone. This applies to everyone and particularly to cases of growing children and in instances where two people sleep together whose ages are widely divergent. The older, stronger child will absorb and sap the strength of the younger one, retarding its growth and development and depleting its physical powers. Each child should sleep alone that it may derive all possible rest and relaxation, during the entire night, necessary to build and restore its body.

The same is true of adults. A more rested, refreshed feeling is obtained when an individual sleeps alone. The vibrations from the other body, while they may afford a feeling of warmth and comfort during cold weather, nevertheless, have the faculty of producing a restless condition which induces insomnia. If an elderly person and one of younger years are sleeping together, the older one seems to draw to itself the strong forces of the younger body, whose vibratory powers are yielded over during the hours of sleep. This has been offered as an explanation of why some mothers who sleep with a daughter who has reached young womanhood, frequently have a very youthful appearance while the daughter looks far more mature than her years warrant. I, personally, am inclined to doubt the reliability of this explanation for it seems hardly plausible that an older body, passing into, if not already in a state of disease and decay, has the power to draw the strength and vitality from a young and healthy body to such an extent that it creates new life and energy in the old one. However, it is entirely credible that we have no voluntary control over ourselves during slumber and since it has been proven that the sub-conscious mind can be influenced during the period of sleep by another's concentrated thought, it may be possible that the bodily powers will also succumb to the octopus-like groping of the older body for health and rejuvenation and energy.

When we sleep alone, we retain all of our body magnetism and draw to ourselves the outside forces necessary to augment our strength. We do not give out our energies and vitality unless another body is there to attract and sap them from us.

Relax before retiring. The body should not be over-taxed with food before retiring—although it is better to eat lightly than go to bed hungry. If the body is fatigued it is advisable to exercise moderately—take 15 or 20 deep breaths and thoroughly relax mind and body before retiring. This will rid the mind of all unpleasant impressions and harassing thoughts of the daily routine and enable you to gain the full benefit of the night's sleep. You will sleep soundly and rest well and awake refreshed and invigorated.

Many people make the mistake of retiring at once when they are extremely fatigued. They make no effort to clear the mind or relax the body, but keep repeating to themselves how tired and exhausted they are. The subconscious mind becomes so impregnated with the thought (and the last thoughts we think before we fall asleep have an important bearing on the sub-conscious) that it is carried through the night and is still with the individual the next morning. He awakens to find himself still tired, worn and enervated. He has received little benefit from his sleep.

Malnutrition due to loss of sleep: Sleep is a food and a complex process which enables the body to feed upon its reserve energy, thereby strengthening and building itself and at the same time storing up more power. Many cases of under-nourishment or malnutrition are due fundamentally to excessive loss of sleep. The digestion becomes chronically impaired through lack of rest and perfect assimilation is impossible; thus, the body already tired and improperly rested, becomes drawn and haggard because it is in no condition to receive and distribute the nourishment taken into it.

Sleep necessary for child's development: The growth of the child depends largely upon its sleeping during the first few months of its life and if that sleep is interfered with through illness, poor care, improper ventilation or any other reason, the child will lose weight and strength. As soon as the disorder is adjusted and the sleep becomes regular and undisturbed, the infant will quickly build and regain the lost weight.

Loss of sleep cause of disease: All disease is the result of a cause and that cause is most frequently a lack of rest and resistance of nerves, which more often than not is due directly or indirectly to loss of sleep. There is quite a differentiation to be made between the few hours rest which the average person *thinks* necessary and the amount of time which is required for real, profound rest to nourish and rebuild the nerves. Perfect slumber induces physical and mental relaxation.

Of course, many people require by nature more sleep than others. Each individual should study his own needs and ascertain just how many hours of sleep he requires to insure a rested and invigorated feeling. If one sleeps too much he will feel dull and stupid, weak and exhausted and will lack ambition to go about his daily work.

One cause of insomnia is an inactive skin which, unable to eliminate properly, produces an irritation of the nerves that induces restlessness and insomnia.

Loss of sleep responsible for many errors: The author has witnessed many miscarriages of justice, due to the jurist's lack of rest, which caused him to be irritable, impatient and lacking in good judgment.

Faulty diagnosis by many physicians could be traced frequently to lack of keen observation and accurate analysis because of a be-fogged brain, hazy from loss of sleep. This may be due, in part, to over-taxation in the physician's work and the handling of cases which demand attention at various hours of the night, all of which takes a heavy toll on the professional man's vitality and unfits him for work which requires hair-line technique and scrupulous precision.

Bedding: The mattress of the bed should always be hard—the pillows, if any, should be small. While a soft bed may feel luxurious and seem conducive to healthful slumber, it is in reality the sponsor of disease. The poisons of the body are eliminated more rapidly at night than during the day; hence the need of more oxygen and the importance of fresh air in the sleeping rooms. If the bedding is soft, the body sinks into it and in this way the circulation of the air over and around the body is checked and interfered with and the poisons are not perfectly carried off. The individual who sleeps in a soft, deep bed with large, fat pillows will have a tendency to puffiness of the body, flabby muscles and unsightly folds in the face, which will eventually become lined with deep creases and wrinkles.

Avoid pillows, as they cause round shoulders and headache. Have the bed clothing light but warm. Most important of all, have the bed arranged so that the sleeper's head is toward the north. This is of very definite importance as it permits the electro-magnetic currents to pass through the body.

Sleep a restorative: If you would have dynamic energy, force and indomitable willpower, see that your body is amply rested and given all opportunity for restoration by at least eight hours sleep each night, and more if it is subjected to any unusual strain.

Those who exert great physical energy need the maximum amount of sleep to enable the body to repair the waste wrought by the day's labor. Persons exercising unusual mental effort require an equal amount of sleep to relax the tension of the mental strain and allow the excess blood to be drawn from the brain and distributed through the body, thus equalizing the circulation.

Sleep is the wonder working agent of nature. All things possessing life must sleep-animals, birds, flowers, plants and insects sleep and even their elements themselves cease their activities at intervals and give themselves over to rest and quiet.

The numerous diseases with which I was afflicted before I rebuilt my body were due to years and years of neglect of both health and body. Lack of attention to exercise, breathing, total disregard of combinations and quantities of food, late hours (I never went to bed before one, two or three o'clock in the morning), all combined to induce chronic and acute diseases which finally affected me to such an extent that I was unable to lie down to sleep because of a continual choking sensation which was due to my enlarged heart. By sitting up I managed to get some relaxation but not enough to call it rest or sleep. If I did attempt to recline I was forced to lie with my hands and arms under my back to regulate the intensity of the pains which racked my limbs and spine.

As a result of the long neglect of body and health I was unable to relax and sleep when I began the regenerating process to overcome my diseases. For six months I went to bed not later than six or seven o'clock but could not go to sleep. By great effort I forced myself to lie quietly and try to relax but, nevertheless I always heard the clock strike the hours and half hours through the night and morning, I was so wakeful and restless.

At last I succeeded in relaxing and was able to sleep finally I reached a point where I could go to bed early;

remain in one position and sleep soundly all night like a child. That was a happy day or rather a happy night in my life. After months of regular, unbroken sleep, my body became rested, the nerves strengthened and filled out and the excruciating pains which had racked my body gradually disappeared. Why? Because the rest and strength derived by the months of regular sleep, exercise, breathing, sun-baths, water and relaxation had built the nerves to a point where they were able to eliminate the diseased conditions and consequently with the passing of disease went the pains which were the manifestation of disease.

This personal experience convinced me beyond question that all diseased bodies are starved for sleep. There are few exceptions to this rule. There are more diseased people than healthy ones and the majority of all bodies lack sufficient sleep to nourish and strengthen the nerves and tissues.

Regeneration of the body cannot be accomplished without balance in all things and while breathing, exercise, sunlight and food are of the most vital importance, the building value and tonic effects of sleep, the great restorative, must never be overlooked.

EXERCISE VS. DISEASE

We go to the theatres, gymnasiums and circuses, where we witness clever acrobatic stunts, exhibitions of gymnastic prowess and performances which require physical agility, skill and daring. We watch with interest, applaud enthusiastically or indifferently according to our mood. Do we ever pause and consider the years of plodding, training, and tiresome practice necessary to build a body capable of performing these parts? Not often. Most of us, preoccupied with business cares, give little, if any, time to exercise. We lead sedentary lives, and we are lazy. We take a street car for a few blocks rather than walk the distance briskly. When we watch and admire acrobats and athletes we all comfort ourselves with the secret conviction that "we could do that if we just got at it." But do we ever get at it? No! From lack of stretching and exercising our muscles, the ligaments become stiff and dry. Our bones crack if we stoop or bend suddenly; we sputter and puff if we run upstairs or hurry for a car, and all because we have long ago abandoned the free and happy movements of childhood, the hops and jumps, wriggles and writhing, reaching and stretching, constant motion and use of all the muscles.

Do you walk quickly? No, lest you appear lacking in grace. Do you run upstairs or down? Not ordinarily—it is undignified. Do you throw your chest out and your shoulders back? No! Because it isn't the fashion—the debutante slouch and the cake-eaters' slump are the smart postures of the moment, and you don't want the world to think you are, by any chance, real, red-blooded he-men and women who don't care a continental for the dictates of fashion but are only interested in surging vitality, robust health and fine, firm bodies. I will tell you right here that if you boys and men would cast aside your cigarettes for good, go in for healthy exercise, develop your bodies and live on the right kind of food, you would be better qualified to *Work* when you work and *Play* when you play, and we should have more successes and fewer failures.

If you girls and women would tear yourselves loose from the fetters of convention, clothe yourselves so that you could take a breath below your collarbone, stretch your limbs in a long, swinging stride, hold your chests up, and by exercise, decrease the fatty tissues of your abdomen until the waist was small and no unsightly fat stomach marred the beauty of your lines, exercise daily and inhale fresh, pure air, we should soon see the last of flat chests, thin arms and board like figures, and view instead the round, plump forms of beautiful, healthy women.

Next to the vicious food upon which our race feeds and depletes itself, the apathetic attitude we assume toward exercise is responsible for the overcrowded state of our hospitals and sanitariums. It is true that in the maelstrom of the commercial world we find little time for the care of our bodies, but a *little time* is all that is required to keep a body healthy and fit. Everyone can spare ten or fifteen minutes a day to exercise and stretch his body. The first few minutes upon arising in the morning are preferable. Always exercise in a room where fresh air is coming in constantly. Move quickly and breathe deeply and you will keep warm through the increased circulation.

Exercise not only to stretch and flex the muscles but to extend and move the bones, and particularly the vertebrae. The closely-woven clothing we wear prevents pores and skin from functioning properly, pampers the body and renders it susceptible to the slightest change of temperature. As you become accustomed to daily exercise your circulation will improve. You will be less liable to contract colds easily, and you will be able to wear lighter clothing.

Guard against too strenuous exercise, however, unless you are accustomed to it. To a beginner the mildest exercises are apt to have a weakening effect, and discretion must be used until the body becomes adjusted. An exercise which consistently benefits one person may result in the death of another, if it is taken up too zealously. The demineralized foods of the present day dry up the tissues, and cause the bones to become so brittle that they may snap under even a slight strain. Exercises should be adapted in accordance with the individual's age, physical condition and diet. Begin gradually, increasing slowly and persistently as the weakening effects of the exercise subside and the body becomes supple.

Due to my persistent efforts in exercising in one manner or another which was responsible for the development of my body to its present state of strength, I found that in order to perfect the health, it was necessary to have exercises which would bring into action all the muscles of the body.

A man may exercise in a way to develop the muscles of certain parts or all parts of his body and still not get exercise which brings into coordination all the muscles of the body and produces health. He may have a beautifully developed body as far as muscular strength is concerned and yet not enjoy perfect health. In his zeal for muscular development he may have overlooked the attention necessary for the perfection of other bodily functions which play an all-important part in the quest for health.

Realizing that all the muscles of the body must be exercised, I was obliged to work out a system of over one hundred and fifty exercises to keep the body properly balanced, supple and pliable.

Exercise is shunned by men and women like a contagious disease. This is a fact. It is a fact which eventually brings about all forms of chronic disorders. I have found and continue to find, that it is impossible to produce a condition of radiant, vital health without following out a system of regular exercise. If you wish to forestall the time of planting yourself in an early grave, loosen up your body every day with some form of good, wholesome exercise or play. Liberate the poisons from your diseased body and brain and your mind will be enlightened with clean, charitable thoughts which are the result of energy and vitality surging through a healthy body.

The abominable long, tight skirts which restrict the movements of the body are again replacing the short, full garment which has found favor with the feminine sex for the past few years. With a long, narrow skirt the freedom of stride is interfered with and instead of stretching the muscles from the ankle to the groin as she walks, the average woman who is fashionably clad walks only from the knee down. The rigid limbs, the small, mincing steps regulated to accommodate the latest mode of dress, indicate a tenseness of body which is in no way conducive to health.

The social dictates by the idiotic autocrats of fashion are responsible for a great many acute nerve and organic diseases. Because of the restrictions enforced on a body trained to adjust its movements to the width and length of hampering clothes, the nerves become atrophied; they are not stretched, exercised or stimulated, so they lose their vitality and premature old age and often paralysis are the result. Any fashion of dress which does not permit the freedom of the limbs should not be tolerated by the human family. This restriction of the leg movement may also be responsible for consumption since it allows no coordination between the lungs and legs. *The shorter the step, the more superficial the breath* Many female disorders have their origin in conditions of this character.

Men and women should discard the time-worn theory and idea that because they have grown up they are any more remarkable than when they were children. On the contrary, their brilliancy has often been dimmed by their growth if it is not actually displaced by stupidity. When they appreciate the fact that after all they are rather stupid and staid and that being only grown-up children, they should enter into things with the same spirit as children, then they will begin to overcome their diseases and promote their own health and happiness.

Parents should romp and play with their children, engage in their exercises and become a part of the child's life. This creates a spirit of harmony in the home, builds the home ties stronger, makes better boys and men and better girls and women, better health and longer life.

Learn to play. Get out of doors. Get back to Nature. Become acquainted with yourself by penetrating the beauties of Nature and learning Her secrets.

Intimate study and understanding of Nature brings a realization of the insignificance of man and his petty pretensions. Nature is profound, and close communion with Her clears the vision and broadens the perspective. Exercise produces Health. Exercise out of doors clarifies the mind as well as the body.

Lack of exercise produces a warped mentality which means perverted thought and subsequent disease. Narrowness, limited and befogged judgment, biased convictions and opposition to all advanced ideas are characteristic of diseased conditions due to lack of exercise, stimulation and all things else which go to make up a perfectly balanced body.

This is a negative state, not a creative one. If a man cannot play, he is mentally unbalanced; he has lost his spontaneity because of disease, either known or unsuspected.

WATER—ITS MEDICINAL ACTION

Water is a food, just as necessary to the body, if not more so, as the everyday meal. One can live on air, water and sleep for weeks at a time with no solid food. He cannot only live but he can also build strength and put on weight. I recently had a young woman patient who decided to go on an extended fast. She did the fasting on her own initiative with the assistance of a healer under whose treatment she had been. She called at my office twice during the first two weeks of the fast, and the change was obvious. Taking nothing but water, exercise and fresh air, her improvement in two weeks' time was so marked that it seemed incredible that she was eating no food. The tissues of the face and neck filled out for the first time since early childhood, as she explained to me, and her face took on a youthful contour and freshness which changed her whole personality. She assured me she felt no fatigue nor hunger whatever.

Water does not, according to the popular conception, enter the bloodstream, wash out its vital properties, thin the blood and cause a general weak and depleted condition to ensue. On the contrary, it flushes the alimentary tract, washes the tiny meshes of the kidneys, which become clogged with the residue of insoluble salts that otherwise gradually accumulate from cooked foods. Water floods the bladder and aids in reducing inflammation of the delicate membranes of the organ. Due to improper diet and general diseased conditions, the urine is often strongly acidic and highly irritating, and when passed will cause a stinging, burning sensation and, in extreme cases, excruciating pain. Hot water taken freely during this period will dilute the urine, greatly relieve the pain and soothe the irritated membranes.

As has been previously mentioned, 75% of the human body is composed of water. Each day everyone should drink one glass of water to every fifteen pounds of his weight if he is eating cooked foods. This is a minimum amount necessary to replenish the daily waste, and it should be taken in addition to whatever watery vegetables and fruits are eaten, for the quantity obtained from the foods is not sufficient to meet the bodily requirements, nor is the action as potent. A large percentage of water is absorbed, softening and stimulating the tissues and quenching the thirst of the infinitesimal cells of the body. The insoluble salts which accumulate from the cooked foods require the consumption of at least one glass of water to every fifteen pounds of the weight because the natural water has been cooked out of the foods and they set up an irritation in the body unless sufficient water has been taken to assist in elimination. People seldom think of drinking water to flush the body. They drink tea, coffee, alcoholic or soda fountain beverages which allay the thirst temporarily but dry up the natural secretions of the body and permit the amassing of insoluble residue from the cooked food.

He who lives upon Raw Food gets water from the vegetables and fruits eaten in their natural state, so he does not require as much water as the person who subsists on cooked food.

In my twenty-five years of practice I failed to find a single person suffering with Pyorrhea who drank enough water. Invariably the individual, when closely questioned, would admit that he or she drank very little water, frequently none at all, depending upon alcoholic beverages, tea and coffee for liquid. To illustrate the action of water, I will cite one of hundreds of cases which I treated with gratifying results. She was a woman nearly sixty years of age, who was brought to me for Pyorrhea treatment. Thin and emaciated, with a withered, leathery skin, her color was of a deep saffron hue, which extended not only all over the face but down the neck, and the ears were parched a and yellow also. Heavy, brown blotches indicated a badly-disordered liver. Her general physical composition proclaimed a melancholy mind, narrow, prejudiced and closed to all advanced thought. Difficulty with a domineering, irascible husband had wrecked her and her daughter, and was responsible for her physical depletion.

Her gums and teeth were badly diseased, and large quantities of pus were being absorbed from the mouth constantly. In conjunction with my surgical treatment for the Pyorrhea I prescribed fourteen glasses of water a day for this patient. Hot water before meals and fresh water between meals and before retiring. This water was taken on a medicinal schedule at prescribed times and with unfailing regularity. The patient was at liberty to drink an additional amount if she chose, but I insisted that she take the fourteen glasses without fail. Within three weeks the liver blotches had disappeared, the skin bleached out, showing a faint pink tint in the cheeks, and even the lobes of the ears became rosy. That woman's entire makeup changed, as well as her personal appearance. Where she had been morose and sullen, she became cheerful, talkative and friendly. Her husband and daughter were amazed at the change. The elimination of the pus from her mouth and the increased amount of water taken into the system effected an astonishing improvement in a remarkably short time. This was one of the most striking responses to the water treatment I have ever seen. The secret of obtaining the greatest benefit from *hot* water is in knowing how to drink it. It should never be taken hurriedly nor gulped down, for water, the same as food, should be mixed with the saliva to promote perfect assimilation. A swallow of the water should be taken into the mouth, the tongue curled up on the sides slightly in a funnel shape, to protect the teeth from the heat, which will shock and congest the nerves and often result in an abscess and subsequent dead pulp. The water should be held in the front of the mouth while the under jaw is moved forward for a second or two. Meanwhile, bring the teeth together with a masticating movement. In other words, chew your water. This movement stimulates the salivary ducts and will cause the saliva to flow readily. After the saliva has blended with the water, the latter is ready to swallow.

These instructions may seem far-fetched and drawn-out, but they have been carefully studied out and practiced over a period of years and their value proved. It requires only a short time to drink in this way, and the results are worth the effort.

Both hot and cold water shock and congest the stomach and teeth, and neither extreme should be taken. A glass of hot water is advisable before meals if cooked food comprises the diet. It is absorbed through the mucous membrane of the stomach, and through its warming and softening influence it stimulates the flow of gastric juices and aids the digestive processes. Water taken before meals should not be boiling hot but only hot enough to cause the ball of the index finger to tingle when immersed in it. This temperature will have no injurious effect but will be found to be very beneficial.

Never drink ice water. Don't drink with meals nor immediately after them.

The inactive fat or bloated individual should take a large swallow of hot water about five minutes before commencing the daily exercise. About every fifteen minutes during the exercises he or she should take another swallow of hot water. The action of the hot water opens the pores, sweats out the poisons and helps in the reduction of adipose tissue. The heat stimulates the functions of the skin and assists in the elimination of the poisons generated from the putrefaction and gas retained in the body. After an extended period of thus exercising regularly and using hot water, the body becomes cleansed and the nerves have a chance to strengthen and build. After the exercises have been completed fresh water should be taken to stimulate and nourish the body.

Hot water is not always advisable. It is to be used during exercising only by people who are fat and bloated and whose bodies carry much poison and waste matter.

For the young athlete whose body is supple, slender and perhaps muscularly drawn, and the nerves thin, the hot water would reduce him too rapidly. The thinning down process would weaken him and dry out the tissues and nerves more than ever.

All exercises should be followed by the internal use of fresh cool water which restores to the tissues the nourishment they need after having undergone the sweating out process of the exercise and hot water, or the exercise alone.

In all treatment for nerve and body building, completely successful results can only be obtained by the copious use of fresh water. I have found that it aids the eliminative processes, promotes the strengthening of the nerves and fills out and establishes a firmness of the tissues. It is one of the most beneficial remedies for curing colds. The average person who is subject to colds does not drink much water. I have never seen people troubled with gall-stones, kidney diseases or hardening of the arteries, who drank sufficient water to perfectly balance the body.

My experience and observation has covered several hundreds of cases. To avail himself of the curative qualities of water, it is necessary to drink on an average of one glass to every fifteen pounds of the weight if the person is living on cooked foods. If he is living on Raw Food, the average may be reduced in proportion to the amount and frequency of the kidney functions as well as the regulation of the diet. About one glass to every twenty or twenty-five pounds should be a fair average if plenty of juicy fruits and water vegetables are eaten.

I think the state or my own health is testimony of the value of water taken internally. At one time I believed as many people still do, that water was made to float ships on. I tried to supplant its value to the body (which is 75 per cent water) by using alcoholic liquors. I drank heavily for a great many years but never included water in the mixtures which I literally poured into my body.

More water internally means fewer operations for kidney stones, gall-stones, stones in the bladder, etc, all of which are calcareous deposits from true excess minerals in the foods which have accumulated because the body was unable to absorb or eliminate them.

Jaundice and liver blotches are further characteristics of people whose bodies are parched for water like thirsty plants withering in a torrid desert.

SUNSHINE—GOD'S ENERGIZER AND DISEASE EXTERMINATOR

Set aside Religious antagonisms and unite in the common search for Health.

Effect on the mind: In the hustle of business affairs and social obligations most people overlook the advantages of sunshine. Yet its curative qualities are miraculous and its reaction instantaneous. If you feel morbid, depressed and lethargic, go out for a walk on a bright, sunny day. Breathe in the clear, cool air, note the blue sky above and the brilliant gleam of the sun's rays on trees and grass. Feel yourself impregnated with a new resolve, observe how your dark, suicidal meditations give way to more optimistic ideas and note how you respond to the cheerful, bright outdoors. Your mood will change in spite of yourself and no matter what your problem, you will find yourself devising a plan to meet and overcome it instead of permitting it to overwhelm you.

On the other hand if you are energetic, high-strung and impatient, go and lie in the warm sand and sunshine on the beach or on a couch in a sunny window. Lie quietly, in the direct path of the sun's rays, for 15 minutes and note the relaxing effect. Your taut nerves will relax, your ambition wane and your impatience recede before a flood of good-natured tolerance which will slowly suffuse you.

The magnitude of all things will diminish and you will be perfectly content to lie there, blissfully contemplating the immensity of space and the immutability of matter. I have sometimes wondered if the warm tropical climate does not account for the sweet and lovable nature of the peaceable tribes of natives that inhabit the Pacific Islands. We are told that they are happy, childlike people, living in a simple, joyous way on the bounties of nature, content to bask in the tropical sunshine and disport themselves in the salt spray of the South Seas.

Until the advent of the white man and the evil influence of his drugs and liquors, these children of nature were robust and beautiful. Their outdoor existence, unhampered by the hideous garments of civilization, developed strong, muscular men and handsome, symmetrical women. With the great outdoors their playground, the fresh fruits and tender nuts their food staples, their lives are ideal and their natures free from the taint of commercialism and race-hatred.

It is a well-known fact that the Europeans who have migrated to these islands and burned their bridges behind them have become just as happy and care-free as the dark-skinned natives. Of course the criticism of the world has been that these individuals have lost their ambition and have become slothful and indolent, but might it not be that, due to the warming, softening influence of the mild, tropical climate, the exaggerated importance of material affairs dissolves into the ether and the idealistic phase of life comes into its own?

Sun and light necessary to all life. The sun energizes the air and soil, and light is essential to vegetable, animal and human life. Neither foliage, grass, animals nor human beings could live without the sun's rays. Recently a lurid tale was brought forth in the newspapers of a girl who had been kept in one room since infancy. Due to some deformity, over which the parents felt greatly humiliated, they had kept the daughter confined in a small room into which practically no light penetrated. When the facts of the case were brought to the authorities and the parents forced to turn the child over to a protective organization, her condition was so feeble that she was unable to stand up but lay helpless and inert, although the mind was fairly active. She told a pitiable story of longing to see the outside world. She had no idea as to what sunshine, blue sky and flowers and grass looked like.

In spite of the child's malformation, which was present at birth, if she had been exposed to the sun and air she would have gathered the strength and vitality which were pitiably lacking. It is even possible that with the assistance of the sun and air, plus a small amount of medical attention, her defect could have been corrected in early childhood. At all events, it is quite certain that if she had been allowed the freedom of the average child instead of being confined to one room for 15 years without ever being taken out, her physical condition would have been much nearer normal than it was, assuming that the deformity was not of a character which would become steadily worse. However, if she managed to survive against great odds in spite of the physical defects and solitary confinement, it is a safe conjecture that she would have developed reasonably sound health under *normal conditions.*

Pallor due to lack of sunlight: Prison pallor is a result of no sunlight. Although the prisoners have light and air, their complexions take on a peculiar waxen color because they are not exposed to the sun for any length of time.

The same is true of office workers.

People whose occupations keep them constantly indoors always show the stamp. They have pallid complexions and dull eyes and in most cases, flabby muscles, and unless they have time to engage in some outdoor sport occasionally and manage to get fresh air and outdoor exercise daily they are apt to be lacking in energy and that radiant vitality which characterizes the perfectly healthy man or woman.

General effects of the sun: Human beings living chiefly outdoors, exposed to the sun, become strong and healthy. Plants thrive in response to the sun's rays—trees and flowers lean toward the sun, bending gracefully to the monarch of the skies. Sun-dried fruits and vegetables are widely recognized for their nutritive merits and the sun-drying process is a commercial proposition which is constantly growing. The sun vitalizes the waters of the sea and the soil of the earth. Its creative power in the growing of vegetation and its therapeutic value are universally acknowledged by scientists and progressive physicians.

The sun as a curative agent. The sun baths of Europe have become famous and many sanitariums and health resorts in America are instituting sun baths as a part of their curriculum. The system of sun-bathing, more technically known as heliotherapy, consists of prolonged exposure of the naked body to the solar rays.

These sun baths date back as far as 1857 European in resorts. The early experiments were confined to exposures of only the diseased parts and as the curative virtues of the sun became apparent, others in the field gradually exposed more of the body. Rollier was the first to expose the entire body. This is done by exposing first the diseased parts for a limited period about three times the first day, a longer period twice on the second day and finally regulating the system until the patient's sun-bath covers a period of about one and one-half hours or two hours. Simultaneously, the body is being gradually exposed to the sun, first the feet, then the legs and so on until the entire body is exposed and the patients can remain out in the open all day without injury.

One process of treatment of laryngeal tuberculosis was practiced successfully by Collet. The patient wears a broad black hat and black spectacles (to prevent serious effects from the sun's rays on the brain and eyes). The patient thus clad sits facing the sun and by means of a special mirror used in examining the throat and larynx, the reflected rays of the sun are directed into the larynx. The periods of exposure are gradually increased until a total exposure of an hour or more is attained.

Sunlight, concentrated and directed through a convex lens of plain glass, has been found to cause destruction of the skin. Gases form under the outer layers of the skin and small explosions occur. This is one method of employing sunlight to cure warts, superficial moles and small benign growths. However, a convex lens must be used as a concave lens will not produce the formation of the gases which are instrumental in eliminating the skin blemishes.

Famous resort for sun and air treatment. Dr. Arnold Rikli established a sanitarium in 1855 Veldes, in the mountains of the Austrian Tyrol. In 1869 this resort came to be known for its light and air cures and from then on Dr. Rikli's experiments with sun and air baths were continuous and successful. The patients at the present time are all required to live, sleep and breathe *entirely* in the open air. They sleep in three-walled thatched-roof cottages— the fourth side of the cottage beings left entirely open. The patients arise at 4 A.M., take a walk in the park, after which they are massaged and made ready for an hour's sun-bath on the roof in the direct rays of the son.

Only a vegetarian diet is served and the eating of raw vegetables and fruits is greatly encouraged. The patients retire at 7 P. M. The men and women are segregated and soon learn to go about all day entirely nude. They take walks in the forests, bask in the sun and get back to nature in the truest sense of the expression. The accounts of those who have visited the resort and taken treatment say that the rejuvenation of mind and body is both remarkable and permanent—as far as any health can be regarded as permanent, which is in proportion to the individual's care of his body.

Dr. Rikli found that the rays of the early morning sun were best, as the sun later in the day was too enervating. Dr. Rikli himself, according to accounts, is mow nearly one hundred years old and is straight as an arrow with browned skin and lustrous eyes.

Benjamin Franklin also believed in the efficacy of air and sun-baths for it is said he wrote and studied at least one-half hour each morning without clothing on.

Effect on nerves. The nerves respond readily to the rays of the sun; they are warmed and soothed; the tension is relaxed so that the gradual healing process begins. Then the nerves recover their vigor, and from the thin, drawn, elongated nerve which characterizes disease, they straighten and fill out to the normal proportions of the healthy nerve. The sun-baths assist more rapidly in building up the resistance of the nerves than any other nonmedical therapy. Indeed, there is no medication which will increase the nerve resistance as quickly and effectively as the sun-rays.

Sun-kissed fruit. It is the sun-rays which tint the cheeks of the peaches, apples, pears and make them so tempting in appearance. Notice the fruit on the shady side of the tree where the sun's rays do not penetrate for long at a time. The fruit there does not have the delicious tint that is found on the sun-kissed product.

Sun-energy. Vegetables and fruits contain sun-energy which when we eat it is transformed into chemical energy; hence the importance of vegetables and fruits in the diet. This accounts for the fact that more physical strength and endurance is often observed in a man who lives on a vegetarian diet than in the meat-eating man. He derives more sun energy from his food than the carnivorous man.

Sun is a natural healer and in combination with pure water and pure air is a powerful disinfectant. Many kind of disease-producing micro-organisms are destroyed by exposure to the strong sunlight.

Sunlight in the home and office: Residences and offices alike should be so constructed as to admit as much sunlight as possible. Where people are fortunate enough to have homes flooded with sunlight, they usually manage to drape the windows sand draw the blinds to shut out most of the light. A dark, gloomy house with the depressing atmosphere of a morgue can be quickly transformed into a cheerful, livable abode, suitable for happy, healthy people merely by raising the blinds and opening the windows. A darkened house is nearly always damp and provides an excellent breeding place for disease since the antiseptic rays of the sunlight are never allowed to penetrate.

Sunlight is the best of tonics. It is a mental as well as a physical stimulant. Don't avoid it—don't shut it out of your home. It is the greatest foe of melancholy and disease—meet it more than half way.

That animal and plant life are dependent on the sun is proven conclusively by the fact that at the equator, where the sun is the hottest, both animal and plant life abound in riotous abundance—while at the polar regions, which are points farthest from the sun, there is no life at all.

Sun-baths not a new fad. The Romans who were enthusiastic sun-bathers, had special sun-rooms or solariums built on as additions to their mansions. With their bodies greased with perfumed unguents to prevent burning, they exposed themselves to the sun's rays for a period each day.

Surgeons have found that the sun is a source of beneficial treatment for wounds, sores and burns. This heliotherapy method was successfully practiced by the German and Austrian surgeons during the Great War.

Discreet use of sun-rays. Sunlight, however, is a dangerous agent if injudiciously applied. Those who live in tropical countries are equipped by nature to withstand the rays of the torrid sun—the animals are supplied with a thick, opaque skin and the human beings are dark-skinned and thick-skulled. The people who live in regions north of the equator are brunettes with dark skins and the farther north and farther from the equator we go, the lighter in coloring we find the people. The brunette heats up more quickly but withstands the ill-effects of the sun better than the blond. The brunette, on the other hand, radiates the heat as soon as he is in the shade and cools off quickly so that he does not suffer from the heat.

A dark vessel attracts heat more quickly than a light one, But a dark one will also cool faster than a light one, as it radiates the heat rapidly. Water will boil more rapidly in a dark kettle than it will in a light one. So while the blonde individual is slower to respond to the sun's heat than the brunette, he stays heated for a longer period and suffers more intensely.

Sun is like radium. It works miracles if used in small quantities, but is extremely dangerous if employed without discretion. Sun is necessary to plant life but too much of it dries and kills the plant. People who visit the tropics are apt to wax enthusiastic over the invigorating effect of the climate at first, but as time progresses they become listless and diseased, their strength sapped by the enervating rays of the sun. The commonest disorders of the hot tropical climate are serious nervous disorders, dysentery, kidney trouble and occasionally a total loss of memory.

It is wise to know both the advantages and disadvantages of the sun baths, as great injury can be done otherwise. Always wear light clothing in hot weather. Light cloth admits the light but reflects the heat while black cloth admits the heat but shuts out the light. Protect the eyes from the glare of the sun during a sun-bath as this glare affects the entire nervous system through the optic nerves.

Sun-baths mean excessive perspiration which drains the water from the body leaving insufficient for the kidneys to dissolve the waste to be eliminated. This water must be replaced at once and a considerable quantity should be taken internally.

Determine how you react in sunlight and regulate your sun-baths accordingly. You will be able to judge in a short time just how much sun agrees with you and what constitutes an excessive dose of sunshine.

BATHING

Water and air are the two most common elements, yet few people know the correct use of either. The people of the cultured upper classes smile in a forced, embarrassed manner when any sly reference to the Saturday bath is made by a low comedian or vaudevillian. Only professional men who are coming in close contact daily with all sorts and classes of people know that the daily bath is shunned by others than those of the tenement districts. Moral, self-respecting citizens clothe themselves and go about their daily duties without the cleansing stimulation of a morning bath. Neither do they seek the solace of a warm bath before retiring.

You may shrug your shoulders in disgust or disbelief—it is true. I have questioned patients who were well-established, active men and women, neat-appearing and intelligent. Various symptoms and often failure to respond to treatment readily would indicate a negligent attitude toward the daily bath. Persistent cross-examination brought out the truth.

Daily bath a necessity for health. For the healthy, active man, woman and child, the daily bath is absolutely essential to health and the immaculate appearance which everyone desires or should desire. No one can look fresh and spotless unless his skin is clear and glowing, and the skin will not take on that smooth, clean texture with a stagnant circulation feeding it. The circulation must, therefore, be stimulated by the daily bath and exercise.

Many doctors and teachers of the present day advocate a bath only infrequently, claiming that the constant application of water to the body undermines the strength and endurance and washes away the natural oils, leaving the skin dry and scaly and the individual more susceptible to chills and cold.

Skin must be cleansed of poison. In extreme cases this is entirely credible, but it is my contention that a man or woman who is at all active and energetic daily eliminates so much poison through the pores of the skin that only constant bathing washes away this poison, cleanses the skin and clears the path for further elimination. Furthermore, unless these poisons are washed from the surface of the body they are re-absorbed into the system, causing disease and lowered vitality.

The odors of an unwashed body are not pleasant. It is a disgusting fact that people visit professional men without being immaculately clean. Often the odor of perspiration is so strong that the consulting room has to be thoroughly ventilated before allowing the next patient to come in. In my own practice it has been a common occurrence to have patients present themselves for dental work with their teeth covered with particles of food, showing that they had not only failed to use their toothbrush after the last meal but had neglected *to* use it for many days previous to the sitting. Incidents of this character so thoroughly disgust a professional man that, were it not for the sake of the few who do earnestly try to care for themselves properly, he would lose interest in his work entirely. It seems incredible that anyone can care so little for himself that he will deliberately compromise his reputation by neglecting the care of his body.

The bodily poisons are thrown out not alone through physical exertion and activity but through the constant use of the brain in thinking and the use of the vocal cords in talking. We know from primary physiology that the slightest movement of the body breaks down millions of cells and this consequent waste must be carried off. Since the skin is an important factor in the process of elimination, we know that some of the poisonous matter is thrown out through the pores, and thus by the slightest elevation of a hand or foot the eliminating functions are again set in motion. It is quite obvious, then, that even an inactive person must be bathed. We have all had the disagreeable experience of trying to keep a sick room wholesome and free from odors even when the disease was not of a character which was notable for any marked impurities. The exudations of the skin are necessarily rancid and poisonous and should never be permitted to accumulate.

Proper bathing. A bath need not be weakening if the temperature is properly regulated and the bath not prolonged. Never have the bathroom stifling hot. It should be thoroughly aerated and afterwards heated to a comfortable warmth to prevent chilling. If the heat is intense and the air impure, the heart action will be so lowered as to cause the bather to become weak and faint.

Only in cases of extreme pain and congestion should a hot bath be resorted to. In instances of this kind a very hot bath is soothing and efficacious in carrying the blood away from the afflicted parts, thereby affording great relief. Cold cloths should be placed on the forehead during the hot bath to prevent dizziness and possible collapse.

The morning bath should follow the daily exercise. Have the water warm enough to accommodate the bodily temperature. Use a coarse turkish cloth or better still, a bath mitt of seaweed. Scrub the body with a pure soap, working up a thick lather. Scrub the body vigorously all over. Many people emerge from a prolonged bath no cleaner than when they entered. They sit and soak themselves awhile, then drag a washcloth lazily around over their bodies and afterwards dry themselves in a listless, haphazard way. These are the people who complain of the weakening effects of a bath. When you bathe yourself—— *bathe* scour the body thoroughly— not so zealously as to irritate the skin but enough to stimulate and cleanse it. Use plenty of soap, but be sure the soap is all rinsed off. Follow this cleansing bath with a quick shower of cool or cold water to close the pores and heighten the circulation. Dry

yourself briskly with a rough towel, don fresh, loose clothing and you will be ready to face the day's problems with
renewed vigor. All this should not require more than 10 or
15 minutes. *Cold plunges inadvisable.* I do not advise cold
plunges. The shock is so great that the kidneys and bladder, as well as the other organs, often become badly
congested, and severe chronic maladies ensue. The shower
should be regulated until it can be turned on cold, but few
constitutions can stand a cold plunge. Many people take a
shower which is cool but not cold. The object is to have the
final spray colder than the bath, to increase the circulation
and prevent subsequent contraction of cold.

Watch your reaction to the cold shower. If you feel
warm and alert after it, experience no chilling sensation or
sniffling, then you react favorably, but if you feel cold and
shivery, if you sneeze and note a congested condition in the
head, if your limbs are inclined to ache and the kidneys
function more frequently than is normal, then the cold
shower is not advisable for you until your physical
strength has been built to a higher point.

Most people who go to the ocean and lakes to swim,
rush out and jump into the water head-first. This is a great
mistake and is often responsible for many diseases which
develop in later life. Before going into deep water to swim,
the body should be gradually chilled down by splashing
the water on the arms, chest and around the region of the
heart. In this way the bodily temperature is reduced, and
when complete immersion takes place the heart is prepared
and the shock is less pronounced.

The hot bath. The evils of the hot bath are many and
great. Pneumonia, influenza, rheumatism and even tuberculosis are frequently the results of extremely hot baths,
which parboil the body—relax and sap the strength of the
nerves and leave the system weak and depleted and so
lowered in resistance that it is susceptible to disease in any
form.

Oil rubs. A very beneficial practice in cold weather is a frequent oil rub. For this purpose use a pure olive oil. After a warm bath before retiring, rub plenty of oil into the entire body, in eluding the soles of the feet. Massage gently and do not rub off the surplus oil. The skin will feel quite oily, but the following morning you will find that all the oil has been absorbed and the body is soft and smooth. Instead of the morning bath, rub the body briskly with a coarse towel and note the stimulating effects. This practice is particularly good in cases of dry, itchy skin and for those who contract colds easily. The olive oil nourishes and builds up the tissues and increases their resistance.

MILK
THE HEALTH AND BODY BUILDER

The value of the "milk-cure" is almost universally recognized by physicians, whose wide experience with neurasthenia, mal-nutrition and chronic alimentary disorders has prompted them to study closely the merits of this assimilable nourishment.

Beauty experts have for years recommended milk baths to keep the skin soft and velvety, but as this is rather a high-priced adjunct to beauty, most of us have been forced to content ourselves with other aids to Venus and Apollo-like physiognomies.

Its food value. Milk and milk products have formed the principal part of the diet of man for centuries back. H. G. Wells, in his "History of the World," in tracing the growth of habit in man down through the ages, writes that milk was first regarded as an unnatural food, but that its evident effect upon life and growth made it permanent. The stalwart tribes which swarmed down through Italy and conquered Rome were fed chiefly upon milk and the produce of the flocks and herds. The peasants of Europe, even when they suffered great privations, and, due to the tyranny of the overlords, were forced to live on black bread and cheese and milk, developed robust bodies and hardy constitutions on this meager fare.

The nutritive merit of milk for undernourished children has been demonstrated in many public schools and charitable institutions of the tenement districts where the underfed children of the poor are given at least a pint of milk each day and in many instances a quart. In the more prosperous neighborhoods the pupils are sold a pint of milk at a very trivial price to encourage wider use of this health-building product.

The propaganda for better health which has been circulated through the schools in the last few years has called the attention of many well-meaning but uninformed parents to a realization of the under-nourished state of their children.

Children who have been put upon a health program whereby they pledged themselves to a stipulated quantity of milk, and an hour of rest each day and a definite number of hours of sleep each night, have increased in weight and strength in a brief time. These children were weighed before entering upon the health program, the weight carefully noted and recorded from time to time and any loss of weight carefully investigated.

Advocated by Health Department. Active campaigns for the increased consumption of milk are being widely advocated by the health authorities of all large cities and many small ones. The former Commissioner of Health of New York City, Royal S. Copeland, now Senator Copeland, issued the statement that he knew of no other food which played such an important part in public health as milk. He also asserted that the *infant mortality rate* for 1921 was the *lowest* the city of New York has ever had, and he said that he felt there was no question but that the increased consumption of pure, wholesome milk was largely responsible for the low death rate.

In Philadelphia a camp organized by the Philadelphia Health Council and Tuberculosis Committee, and largely supported through the co-operation of the Department of Welfare, has been increased from a capacity accommodating 50 children in 1920 to 1,000 in 1922. These undernourished children, most of whom have been sufferers from tuberculosis, are lined up twice a day for milk service. Each child receives a complete physical examination before admission to the camp, and that, with the subsequent records of weight and general improvement, is filed in the camp office.

Sleeping in tents, wholesome food, exercise and a bountiful supply of milk, 165 quarts of which are donated daily by the Interstate Dairy Council, returns all of these happy little campers to the city in a vastly improved condition and restores many of them to perfect physical trim.

Surely Health Departments, Departments of Welfare and other civic as well as charitable organizations, would not liberally donate and encourage the investment of money in milk for the little diseased underlings of the crowded cities, unless the statistics proved beyond a doubt the worth of that investment.

The yearly milk bill of a leading hospital in London averages over $80,000. These figures provide a reasonable estimate of what scientists and physicians think of milk as related to the treatment of disease.

The milk treatment and its effective *cures* embrace almost every conceivable disease. Acidity, albuminuria, anemia, arthritis, asthma, auto-intoxication, biliousness, Bright's disease, constipation, dyspepsia, mild skin eruptions, gall-stones, goiter, heart disease, insomnia, neuritis, nervous prostration, sciatica and gastritis are only a few of the diseases which respond readily to a milk diet. The milk-cure is also most efficacious in correcting the cocaine, morphine and tobacco habit.

Milk supplies all needs. Milk is rich in the *vitamins* necessary to life, and it contains the salts necessary to build every part of the body. Iron, potassium, phosphorous, sodium, lime, magnesium, flourin, etc.—about twenty elements in all are contained in milk. Because of an internal secretion contained in milk and the percentage of iron it carries, it is invaluable in the treatment of thyroid or lymphatic gland disorders. Grave's disease or goiter is one manifestation of a lack of iron in the system, and although milk contains a small amount of iron, it would appear that

it is in a form which is exceptionally favorable to assimilation and sufficient to supply the requisites of the human
system.

There are those in the medical profession who refer to
the fallacies of the milk cure, but it seems only reasonable
to suppose that these physicians, who are in the minority,
are either biased and negative to new ideas, or their
experience has been extremely limited.

The necessity of milk for expectant and nursing
mothers and growing children cannot be too greatly
emphasized, as it is an important factor in building teeth
and bones, as well as flesh.

Puny, sickly children and adults have developed
robust, vigorous health when milk was made the principal
part of their diet for an extended time.

Cure for venereal disease. There are several reports on
record of syphilitic and gonorrheal cases having been
completely cured on a milk diet. After an extended fast and
prolonged and exclusive milk diet, the Wasserman tests
gave a negative reaction. Of the curative and building
properties of milk, this leaves little room for doubt. In each
instance, fine physical bodies were built up and a powerful
manhood developed where formerly the individual was of
mediocre development and doubtful ability.

The reports and statistics submitted by physicians
who do extensive experimenting in milk treatment, do not
attempt to explain whether the beneficial action of milk is
due solely to its great nutritive qualities or to some occult
medicinal power unknown to man.

Chyle is the milky fluid which is found in the lacteals
of the intestines after digestion. It is Lymph plus digested
food. Lymph is a transparent, slightly yellow fluid of alkaline reaction which fills the Lymphatic vessels. It is
generally assumed that because of milk's resemblance to
chyle it is so easily assimilated. Milk absorbs into the lymphatic circulation and thence into the bloodstream.

Some authorities maintain that *diseased kidneys* cannot only be appreciably improved but in many instances can be actually *restored* to perfect condition on a milk diet. Serious cases of *Bright's disease* have responded favorably and permanently to the milk cure.

Milk as a heath medium is presumed to have valuable influence as a preventive of some diseases and a cure for others. It is rich in the much discussed vitamins which are essential to life and health.

Specialists in milk cures tell us of immediate reaction to the milk cure. A cure, of course, is taken with the patient confined to bed. One authority states that within three to twelve hours the heart action is accelerated, the pulse increased and the functioning powers of the skin greatly stimulated. This is due to the increased amount of blood which is created in a natural, normal way by the stomach and intestines acting upon the easily-assimilated food in the form of milk. One of the striking features of the milk cure is the prompt return to normalcy of the pulse, and it may be very high or very low with either a slow or rapid heart.

Have you ever considered that a child's body is built on milk? That the foundation of its entire life is laid during those early months when milk is the sole and indispensable factor of its diet? That it builds flesh, bone, hair and teeth on milk alone? That it has all of these developments before any other food forms a component part of its regular diet? *Malnutrition* would not undermine our vitality and sap out our very lives if milk were substituted for the quantities of tea, coffee, alcoholic and soda fountain beverages which are annually consumed by the people.

The Author's Personal Experience with Milk in Building Health

I am a great advocate of milk for the reason that I lived for one whole year upon milk, water, air and sleep, the only addition being fruit juices. I know the value of milk. My diet at the present time consists largely of milk. By that I do not mean that I exclude other foods, but in proportion to the amount of other foods which I eat, milk is the predominant element of my dietary. I now drink milk where I formerly drank tea, coffee and alcohol.

After having been practically given up to die by my physicians and having suffered excruciating pains for eighteen years, from which I was able to obtain no relief, it was at this point that I determined to turn the tables in my own favor, by learning the secrets of my body which would be instrumental in building my health.

Milk, along with air, much sleep and light exercises (which I was only able to practice while lying down on a bed), was an important factor in effecting the improvement and cure which were finally achieved. Naturally, I cannot now forsake nor neglect to cite, the remarkable curative food which built me to the state of health I possess at the present time.

Milk is, in my opinion, the only medium through which perfect regeneration of the body can be obtained.

I would advise those who are seeking Health and wish to rebuild themselves, to become thoroughly conversant with the surpassing value of milk which carries all the elements necessary to build the body. Milk is the only thing which builds babies. If milk will build the body and health of a baby it will regenerate our bodies and lost vitality since after all we are only grown up babies.

VITAMINS

Vitamin—from the Latin, vita, meaning life,
and minum, meaning small—small life.

Vitamins are a class of substance the exact composition of which is yet unknown. They exist in minute quantity in the *natural* foods, in the *uncooked* foods, in the hull, or outside covering, of the grains and in the peelings of fruits and vegetables. The vitamins are necessary to perfect nutrition and growth, and without them life cannot be sustained. The absence of vitamins from the diet produces what is known to the medical profession as deficiency diseases, beri-beri, scurvy, leprosy and rachitis.

These diseases are most prevalent in the tropics and the orient, where polished rice and various starchy and canned foods comprise the greater part of the diet, with a dearth of greens and juicy, fresh vegetables.

Demineralized foods: The highly refined foods of the present time not only fail to nourish because they have been divested of their life-giving elements, but they are actually injurious to the point of being dangerous. The popular processed cereals, white flour, rice and granulated sugar have been so highly refined and bleached by the time they reach the market that they are completely demineralized and carry no nourishment whatever. They merely act as irritants to the stomach and alimentary tract, generating acids which infiltrate the bloodstream and absorb the alkalinity so that the blood, instead of carrying alkaline nourishment to the tissues, supplies them with an excess of acid which dries up the natural secretions of the joints, and results in acidosis and many diseases, such as arthritis deforming, rheumatism and neuritis.

The boiling of foods destroys a large percentage of the vitamins, and a temperature above the   boiling point kills them. It has been stated, that our modern diet is so deficient in vitamins—in other words, that we eat so much cooked, devitalized food that it is only the occasional plate of salad, stalk of celery or raw onion, all of which are rich in vitamines, that sustains our lives at all. This may seem an exaggeration, but if we consider that no animal can live long on cooked foods, that animals as well as human beings must have organic food materials, that animals fed on cooked food until they are near death will be quickly restored to health through the administration of small quantities of vitamins, it is conclusive evidence that the diet upon which we subsist is certainly not a correct one. Out of nearly 100,000 species of animal life, human beings are the only species that rely upon inorganic (or cooked) food for sustenance. And human beings are constantly ailing, whereas animals in their native habitat live healthy undisturbed lives until their allotted period expires.

A normal supply of organic mineral salts is the crying need of the populace, and inorganic salts cannot meet this demand. Organic salts carry the vitamins which are essential to human life.

Vitamin seems to be an all-inclusive term, the exact meaning of which is rather elusive. It is assumed that vitamins are a mysterious element contained in the mineral salts. If we refer to the deposit which mineral salts throw off in the system, as an ash, the meaning becomes clear at once. An ash is what remains after a product has been burned, and the ash deposited in the system after food has been burned in the human incinerator, the stomach, is similar to the ash found in the hearth after the burning of wood. After the burning of whole wheat, whole corn, natural rice and milk, the residue is similar to an ash. This burning, performed as a laboratory experiment and followed up by an analysis of the ash deposit, discloses that the ash is composed of compounds of iron, lime, potassium, phosphorus, sulphur, magnesium, silicon, sodium. However, the chemical change effected by the heat produces an ash which is vastly different in structure from the ash which is evolved from the digestive incineration carried on in the stomach. Hence it is easily understood what a ridiculous idea it is to suppose that we can buy our vitamins at the corner drug store and rebuild our bodies on these marvelous rejuvenating vitamin tablets or liquids. Foodstuffs contain no ash, but the mineral salts are thrown off in the system in the form of an ash. However, if the foods are highly refined and demineralized, they will deposit no ash in the system and will convey no nourishment to the body.

Little or nothing definite is known concerning vitamins. They are a mysterious and seemingly mythical something about which no tangible evidence has been submitted. They supposedly carry proteins, carbohydrates, fats and mineral salts. The foods which are almost universally neglected and omitted are those which carry the much-needed mineral salts. Few people languish from a lack of proteins, carbohydrates and fats, but it is a rare thing to find an individual whose diet is so well balanced as to include a rational amount of the mineral salts plus the three constituents first named.

Iron, potassium, calcium rank first among the organic salts essential to body building— iron for blood, potassium for muscles and nerve-tissues, and calcium for the bones and teeth.

Iron oxide corrects internal respiration and builds the hemoglobin or red corpuscles of the blood. The coloring matter of plants is derived from the iron contained in the soil in which they grow; hence the color of the blood is dependent upon a good supply of red blood, and although a reserve of lime and phosphorus is held in the body, practically no iron is stored up; hence it is essential that great care be exercised in selecting foods which amply supply this indispensable element.

Raisins contain iron in its most assimilable form. Then in the order of their percentage of iron come lettuce, spinach, leeks, strawberries, asparagus, radishes, apples, prunes, cherries and blackberries.

Potassium is found in lettuce, cauliflower, cucumber spinach, potatoes, olives, watermelon, cherries, pears, prunes, grapes and apples.

Calcium may be obtained in spinach, cabbage, lettuce, radishes, carrots, cucumbers, watermelon, strawberries, figs, prunes, grapes, pears and apples.

Chemical analysis has established beyond question that everything required for the sustenance of man is contained in vegetables, fruits, nuts, raw grains and milk, and since the vegetables and fruits carry the organic alkaline salts which are so valuable in neutralizing the acid wastes of the body in addition to their paramount functions of building blood, bone, muscle and nerve tissues, and nuts, milk and raw grains contain the essential proteins it is quite obvious that perfect health can be maintained on all of these if they are eaten in their natural, uncooked state.

To insure getting your quota of these mysterious vital vitamins, eat more raw vegetables, fruits, rnuts, raw grains and milk. Eat more fruits, less pastry, more raw foods and less of the cooked, mushy starches, for it is only the raw foods which carry 100% vita-mines.

FASTING

Where one person dies of starvation, thousands go to an early grave from over-feeding. At the suggestion of a fast, or even a greatly-restricted diet, the average person is convinced that his days are numbered. In many cases they *are* numbered unless he employs dietetic discretion and gustatory restraint.

Most people think of death from starvation as being close at their heels if they miss even one meal, and they look with astonishment and disapproval upon the person who omits breakfast or lunch.

Of all the organs of the body, the stomach is perhaps the most over-worked and long-suffering, for it is no sooner emptied than it is filled again, and frequently the re-filling process begins before the evacuation takes place.

Due to this constant strain of over-taxation, the stomach often becomes prolapsed, functionally disturbed and generally inactive. The results are, innumerable diseases, loss of health and, not infrequently, death can be directly traced to some fundamental stomach disturbance.

The stomach needs an occasional rest. Normally it is evacuated in from five to seven hours. How many people permit the stomach to empty itself of one meal before they eat anything else? Many people are eating constantly, never allowing the stomach any respite whatsoever.

Many minor disorders can be quickly cleared up by fasting. Indigestion, constipation, gas, colds and headache can be speedily relieved by a few days complete fast or a diet of fruit juices and water, accompanied by exercise and deep breathing.

The body is thus permitted to eliminate more freely since it is not congested and overloaded. The poisons and gases are expelled, the inflated tissues are relieved, the distended organs assume their normal position, and the tense muscles and overstrained nerves gradually relax and build.

Occasional fasts are of the greatest value. Both mind and body are benefitted, and new vigor and purpose accrue to the faster. Prolonged fasts are advisable in acute conditions, but always with the approval of a physician who is thoroughly conversant with the patient's case, his strength and endurance, and understands scientific fasting and natural curative methods.

Fasting does not impair the strength, but on the contrary it increases the faster's power and energy *provided* that the physical condition is such that it warrants a fast.

Fasting, to be successful, has to be regulated according to the acute, nervous or chronic condition of the patient. All cases cannot be put on a rigorous fast with no preliminary preparation. Many people are so terribly impoverished and so badly depleted that to put them upon a complete fast will mean certain death. If the individual is weakened by disease and extreme fatigue, he must first be built up with rest, sunshine, light exercise, deep breathing, water and oil.

It has been my experience that to receive the real benefit of fasting the body must be built up to a resistive point so that when the fasting process begins the body has sufficient strength and energy to stand the breaking down of the cells and the elimination of poisons. Some people are so undernourished that their bodies have been literally fasted for years through being nerve-starved.

I have found alternate fasting to be very beneficial in some acute and many light chronic cases. If the patient is broken down and unable to stand the straight, consecutive fast, he can fast one day, eat the next and fast again the following day, and so on. If he wishes, he may fast one day; the next day he may drink fruit juices and buttermilk or eat fruits or a light vegetable salad, and the third day go back to the fast. By this alternate fasting system much good can be accomplished. The body can be cleaned of its impurities and the overworked digestive organs given a thorough rest.

Occasional fasts which are prolonged for several days or a week are of great assistance where the body requires a complete cleansing, as in cases of indigestion, dyspepsia, constipation, headaches and extreme nervousness.

In all cases of fasting, sleep is an important substitute for food. Sleep nourishes and rests the nerves and tissues and builds strength of mind as well as body. The exercise should be light and may be taken in bed if necessary. Sunshine and fresh air must be taken in large quantities; both stimulate and revivify. Deep breathing burns out the impurities and oxygenates the blood. Not less than ten deep breaths of pure, fresh air should be taken every hour during a fast. Constant stimulation and purification is thus afforded the lungs, blood and tissues. The bowels must be kept open with a high-grade mineral oil and should move every day for the first few days. Constipation may occur after a few days, followed by an attack of dysentery. These peculiarities are due to functional conditions and can be regulated according to the case. Water oxygenates the tissues, cleanses the body and promotes elimination. Contrary to most convictions, it does not wash out and thin the blood. Water is a food and not only cleanses but nourishes the body and assists the cells in disposing of their poisons.

During a prolonged fast the patient should refrain from all conversation and thinking. Talking saps the vitality of the nerves, making them highly excitable and irritable. This condition arrests the patient's progress and should be avoided. All mental effort should cease, and the patient should allow his mind to be disturbed by nothing. He should *visualize* constantly the state of health which he wishes to attain and never allow that mental picture to be replaced by any other.

Great care must be exercised in breaking an extended fast. If large quantities of food are eaten immediately, great pain and possible collapse may result. The fast should be broken gradually, increasing the quantity as the quantity of a child's food is increased, in proportion to its gain in strength. Fresh popcorn without salt or butter is recommended by some for breaking a fast, but I cannot personally vouch for its merits.

Fasting is the only means of effecting a perfect cure of practically all diseases. Most diseases are greatly aggravated by the continuous ingestion of food, and few, if any, fail to respond to a scientific fast, accompanied by rest, sunshine, fresh air, water and oil and followed by a proper diet of foods which contain 100% nutrition.

As has been stated, however, the prospective faster must be built up to a high point to enable him to gain best results from the fast.

There is no question but that scientific fasting eliminates the bodily poisons, adipose tissue, and breaks down destructive cells. If properly and scientifically carried out, the fast is a means of acquiring complete rejuvenation and vigorous, robust health.

SUGAR

The almost exclusive use of white sugar along with white flour constitutes one of the greatest dietetic curses of the age.

The ordinary white sugar, whether in granulated, loaf or pulverized form, is an acid-bleached extraction of the pure cane sugar, which has been put through such a refining process that it retains no more of the characteristics and attributes of the original product than does an angel-food cake to the whole grain wheat from which it is evolved after the wheat has been milled, processed and refined to conceal its natural identity.

White sugar is an acid producer.

It is an artificial commodity and has most injurious effects on the body.

Sugar in its natural state, produced by the body's action on vital foods, is essential to the bodily functions. Sugar is an indispensable product to the system. It generates heat, which in turn creates energy and power.

However, only one-tenth of one percent of sugar can be absorbed into the bloodstream. All in excess of that amount means the breaking down of vital organs.

The function of the pancreas is to restrict the excess absorption of sugar into the bloodstream. Inordinate consumption of sugar in beverages, pastries, candies, cakes, ice cream and other soda fountain drinks which seems a characteristic of the American people, that supersedes similar tendencies of all other nations, overtaxes the pancreas and calls for more strenuous action on the part of the liver, kidneys, lungs and skin to dispose of the excess sugar.

Medical science has established the fact that all excess sugar is eliminated through the kidneys. Thus kidney diseases and disorders are becoming more and more prevalent in proportion to the universal consumption of sweets.

The saliva of man contains a ferment which converts the starches of potatoes, rice, corn, beets, carrot, etc., into the natural sugar required for the body's use. By increasing the amount of sugar in the body the salivary glands are deprived of their normal activity in producing the ferments which convert the starches to sugar.

In many of the commercial sweets and beverages, glucose is substituted for sugar. According to a reliable estimate, about 80% of the glucose manufactured from corn is distributed to bakers, confectioners, jam and jelly manufacturers, the purveyors of synthetic fruit juices and syrups.

An excessive ingestion of refined sugars, starches and glucose is believed to be the cause of diabetes. All evidence and observation strongly substantiates this theory. At all events, diabetic conditions are greatly aggravated if these products be continuously included in the diet and speedily ameliorated if they are excluded.

Supposedly the impairment of *pancreatic* functions induces *diabetes.* The pancreas when in a normal healthy state appropriates lime and potassium salts, which constitute part of the chemical composition of the pancreatic secretions. Glucose has an affinity for these salts, and the theory has been extended that the condition of glycosuria (excess glucose in the system), which constitutes diabetes, is responsible for the loss of lime and potassium salts in the pancreas and its consequent impaired functioning The pancreas is thereby weakened and unable to offset the attacks of the excessive glucose or check its access to the bloodstream.

Glucose, combining with the lime and potassium salts, form compounds which in solution are said to have a remarkable tendency to absorb oxygen.

Thus a diabetic individual suffers a deprivation of oxygen along with his other miseries.

Sugar and calcium have a marked affinity for each other.

Calcium is an essential mineral salt   Without it we could not build bones and teeth. People who have strong teeth are generously supplied with calcium. Those whose teeth are weak lack calcium, either through a natural deficiency or because the quantities of sugar and glucose which they consume attack the calcium of the tissues. The tissues, requiring calcium, appropriate that mineral from the blood, and the blood in turn is forced, in order to maintain its minimum of calcium, to abstract the calcium from the teeth. Hence, the strength of the teeth is undermined, and they become chalky and brittle.

It is the author's firm conviction, arrived at after years of research and observation, that the immunity which should be the birthright of every child is destroyed by the mother's diet during the period of pregnancy. The white sugar contained in pastries, puddings, cakes, candies, jellies, jams, ice-cream, etc., along with other demineralized products, forms an excess acid which cannot be neutralized by the secretions of the body. These acids attack and *soften the bones,* undermine the strength and vitality of the mother, who transmits to her child a predisposition to weakness which makes the child susceptible to such diseases as *infantile paralysis, spinal meningitis, tuberculosis, anemia, diabetes* and other diseases deadly to child growth and development.

Many children who appear plump and healthy are really *under-nourished* and *waterlogged*. Like salt, an excess of sugar in the system requires water to hold it in solution, and thus the tissues become distended with water, and the weight increases as more sugar and glucose are eaten.

The health of all children and prospective mothers is endangered so long as they continue to live upon demineralized products and white sugar.

The conditions which arise as a result of this diet can be overcome and offset by changing the cooked diet to one comprised of vital nourishing foods which contain the highest possible percentage of nutrition and will not only keep the prospective mother strong and healthy during pregnancy and fortify her against the distressing aftermath, but will enable her to endow the child with the physical strength and power which spells immunity from the fatal diseases to which weak, undernourished and congenitally-depleted babies fall heir.

Honey should be substituted for sugar. Honey, maple sugar, dates, figs and raisins are concentrated, natural sweets and heat producers.

Most marketable honey is strained and sold in liquid form. It is more economical for the bee keeper to extract the honey and use the combs over and over than to put the bee to the exertion of rebuilding combs.

All honey granulates unless heated for thirty minutes or more at 160 degrees Fahrenheit.

Granulated honey is just as pure as liquid honey.
Honey builds and nourishes.
White sugar breaks down and destroys.
Honey does not create acid.

White sugar causes fermentation and the generation of acid, which softens the bones and destroys the nerve fiber.

HAIR

Thick lustrous hair is a distinctive mark of beauty for a woman and it certainly enhances the appearance of a man.

The hair protects the head and scalp from extreme thermal changes and preserves the brain and nerve centers from shocks, injuries and irritation from external influences.

It is an organ of touch, since it is extremely sensitive and gives warning of danger. This is evidenced by the hair standing erect when touched, also standing on end from fear, anger, etc.

It is a great advantage to retain the hair and it should be given the greatest consideration.

All diseases of the hair and scalp are directly due to the conditions of the system and the hair reflects the state of health. Diseases of the scalp and loss of hair are only expressions of bodily ailments. The color, luster, oil, dryness and brittle quality of the hair are all influenced by the systemic conditions.

Any disease which impairs the vitality of the body has a direct effect upon the hair. A poisoned bloodstream carries little or no nourishment to the scalp and the circulation being diminished by the general nerve conditions, the cells of the scalp are depleted. The vitality of the hair is endangered and unless the conditions are noticed soon enough to correct them, the papilla, which fosters the hair, dies and the hair falls out.

Women have deeper hair follicles than men and a greater supply of sebaceous glands which afford more nutrition.

Baldness in old men is due to a thickening of the scalp and a weakening of the blood supply to the hair roots.

According to Dr. R. W. Muller, each hair should be regarded as a plant growing in a garden, which is the scalp. The bloodstream fertilizes the hair plant and keeps it healthy and strong.

The circumstances which determine the life of a hair are not known.

The eyelashes last about 130 days and an individual hair on the human head lasts from one to six years.

The hair grows faster by day than by night; in warm weather than cold, and faster in middle age than any other time.

Thermal extremes are supposed to induce the growth of the hair more rapidly than moderate temperatures, although the exact reason for this is not given. The theory might be advanced that extreme cold weather stimulates the circulation to the scalp and induces the hair growth while extreme heat has an incubating effect.

The chemical composition and constituents of the hair according to Waldeyer are as follows: 100 parts of hair contain from .5 to .7 parts of incombustible materials. This contains 23 per cent alkaline sulphates, 2 to 10 per cent oxide of iron and 40 per cent silica. Dark hair contains more iron than light hair.

Analysis of the hair substance proves it to be composed of

Carbon	50
Oxygen	20.85
Hydrogen	6.36
Nitrogen	17.14
Sulphur	5

Fair hair contains less carbon and hydrogen and more oxygen and sulphur.

Brown hair contains more carbon and a small amount of oxygen and sulphur.

White hair of aged people contain quite an amount of bone earth or phosphate of lime.

The percentage of nitrogen is about the same in all hair.

The oils of the hair vary in color according to the color of the hair.

The papilla which fosters the hair and builds new hair cells is the connecting link between the blood and nerve supply of not only the general circulation, but the nervous system and the hair.

Causes of baldness. Loss of hair and baldness may be due to catarrh, mental disorders, worry, injuries, friction, skin diseases, nervous diseases, tuberculosis, typhoid, venereal diseases, over or under-functioning of the sex organs, blows, bruises, dyes, bleaches, excessive shampooing, injurious tonics and salves and cure-alls for itching scalps and falling hair.

Physicians claim that the taking of mercury and the iodides seriously affects the hair. Venereal diseases destroy the pigment and cause the hair to turn white.

Thallium acetate which is given to arrest the progress of tuberculosis, causes the hair to start falling out within from two to eight days after its use.

Wounds, burns, fright, hot and cold sweats and the treatment for them causes loss of vitality and death of the hair.

There is a definite connection between the genital organs and the sebaceous glands which nourish the scalp. The normal sex functions stimulate the activity of the sebaceous glands and the over-functioning of the genital organs has a depleting effect on the sebaceous glands of the scalp, drying their secretions and exhausting the vitality *of* the hair.

Arthritis is a disease of the joints, which impinges the nerves and diminishes the circulation. It is one of the greatest causes of destroyed pigment, producing white hair and causing baldness.

Carbuncles have an idiosyncrasy for erupting on the back of the neck near the hair border.   They spread and enlarge very rapidly, are accompanied by a high fever and destroy the hair border.

Dryness and dandruff are indications of scalp trouble. The itching resulting from these conditions provokes excessive scratching The scalp becomes irritated from the scratching and friction and infection frequently occurs.

Ring-worm, hardening of the arteries, scar-letina, headaches, ear-troubles, infected teeth, malnutrition, all toxic diseases and all habits and foods which change the functions of the sebaceous glands are responsible for scalp conditions.

Incidental causes of baldness and hair trouble. Bad combs, brushes, pulling hair with combs, accidental loss of hair due to burning of hair with chemicals and caustics.

Vegetable parasites and microbe parasites produce conditions which cause baldness.

Seborrhea, which is presaged by itching, is a distinctive disease of the scalp and causes the death of the hair cell and loss of the hair.

Baldness is a manifestation of the death of the hair due to insufficient normal circulation and nourishment to the papilla, the hair mother.

With increased weight there is a decrease of hair. The excessive eating of cooked foods inflates the body and builds adipose tissue. The nourishment which should be distributed through the system and to the scalp is employed in building fatty tissue and consequently hair is deprived of its rightful sustenance.

Resorcin, which is an ingredient of many tonics, causes seborrhea and baldness.

Dandruff is a flaking of the scalp the same as the scaling of the skin of the body. Dandruff is caused by irritation to the scalp.

Hats deprive the hair of air and cause it to fall. False hair, too many hair pins and combs should be avoided. Curling, waving and crimping with metal curlers and hot irons dries and breaks the hair.

Manifestly, the real protection of the hair and the treatment for diseases of the scalp lies not in the various ointments, tonics, salves and various applications sold for the purpose, but in attention to the foods which are fundamentally the causes of all diseases of the body, including those of hair and scalp.

A diseased scalp is an indication of impurities in the bloodstream and like skin diseases, no results are obtained unless the cause of the trouble is reached.

The bloodstream which carries nourishment and stimulation to the scalp and hair must be purified by the use of nourishing, wholesome foods which build the body and restore the vitality to the hair.

All nervous diseases and diseases which in any way affect the nutrition of the body have a seriously depleting effect upon the scalp and cause the hair to die and fall. Special attention to the foods which carry the greatest nourishment to the body is the paramount consideration. Since the analysis of the hair proves it to be composed of carbon, hydrogen, nitrogen, oxygen, sulphur and iron it is obviously necessary to eat the foods which will supply the system with these minerals.

Cooked foods cannot do this for most of the minerals are boiled out and drained off.

Raw foods carry the highest percentage of minerals obtainable.

In the order of their percentage of the specified mineral, the following foods are tabulated:

Iron. Raisins, lettuce, spinach, leeks, strawberries, asparagus, radishes, apples, prunes, cherries and blackberries.

Sulphur. Horseradish, spinach, cauliflower, cabbage, radishes, asparagus, cucumbers, onions, potatoes, figs.

Silicon. Lettuce, oats, wheat, spinach, asparagus, barley, horseradish, strawberries, cucumbers, onions and cherries.

Carbohydrates. (Foods containing hydrogen, oxygen and carbon.) Potatoes and rice, honey, brown sugar, raisins, figs, dates and prunes, cereals, wheat, rye, oats, carrots, peas, string beans and beets.

Foods containing carbohydrates are composed of pure starches, as potatoes and rice; concentrated sweets, honey and brown sugar, raisins, dates, figs and prunes; mixed starches, as cereals, wheat, rye, oats, carrots, peas, string beans and beets. The last group is composed mainly of starch but contains also some protein and possibly a small amount of fat and some minerals.

Neither the electric dryer nor any hot air should be used on the hair.

Dry hair should not be washed often and alkaline substances only should be used on it. The best preparations for dry hair are made of olive oil, oil of sweet almonds, Vaseline and beef marrow, to which aromatic essences may be added. Dry hair is often due to anemia, dyspepsia, malnutrition, utero-ovarian and nervous troubles. The first step is to treat the general condition. The second to improve the tone of the scalp and stimulate the growth of the hair cells.

In cases of extremely oily scalps, the hair should be washed often with Hebra's alkaline soap or soft soap, and the use of *preparations* of alkalines (borate of soda, bicarbonate of soda) is also indicated.

According to Broqc, preparations of ammonia are excellent. It is also advisable to powder with inert powders, oxide of zinc or starch and orris root powder, leaving it on for several hours and then brushing out.

Scalps which perspire freely should be washed often with lukewarm water, diluted with alcohol or aromatic vinegar.

Cutting and singeing are of no value in stimulating the growth of the hair. Cutting retards the growth, singeing dries and splits the hair.

Oil of pure vaseline, pomades with sulphur and tar are advocated for the treatment of dandruff. Never apply alcoholic tonics to a dry, scaly scalp.

Treatment of the hair. The scalp should be manipulated lightly with the tops of the fingers or the palms of the hands, always moving it in a rotary movement. With the palms of the hands pressed against the sides of the head, the scalp should be moved gently and pushed into folds. This keeps it loose and prevents it from becoming hidebound, a condition nearly always present in cases of heavy loss of hair. The manipulation should be very light and not enough to irritate the scalp.

Moderate use of a good brush and comb on the HAIR, not the scalp, keeps the hair smooth and lustrous. Many people comb and brush the scalp vigorously, believing that they are stimulating it when in reality they are producing irritation.

Never use great force in handling the hair. The scalp is not only irritated and injured but the hair itself is broken off.

Head breathing is absolutely essential to a healthy scalp. There can be no life where there is no oxygen. Head breathing oxygenates the scalp, increases the circulation and stimulates the hair follicles. Too frequent washing changes the color of the hair and destroys its vitality. It should be washed when the scalp is dirty, about once a month. Simple lotions for shampooing are:

1.   Hebra's alkaline soap (fluid) or tincure of green soap—
     (Muller).
2.   Boiled water (500 grammes) with the yolk of a beaten
     egg—(Muller).
3.   Lime water (500 grammes) with the yolks of three
     eggs—(Jackson).

To properly shampoo, wet the head thoroughly with
warm water. Make a thick lather on the hands with a soap
and rub vigorously into the scalp. Rinse out thoroughly
with warm water and finish with cool water—not cold.
Rub the hair dry with hot bath towels, changing them as
quickly as they moisten.

Dont's and Preventives

Don't wash the hair too frequently.

Don't exercise too much vigor in massaging, brushing
and combing.

Don't neglect conditions of dandruff, itching, extreme
oiliness and dryness. If local care is ineffective, consult a
specialist arid follow his directions.

Don't curl, crimp, snarl or otherwise injure the hair.

Don't fuss with your hair and scalp unnecessarily.
Give both a rest.

Change the style of hair dressing. Adherence to one
arrangement influences the growth and direction of the
hair and makes it fall out.

Men should remove their hats whenever possible,
even carry them on the street occasionally, thus enabling
the hair to breathe.

Women should never sleep with their hair coiled up. It
should be let down at night, brushed gently and braided in
several braids if extremely thick. If not too thick, it is
advisable to let the hair hang loose and allow it to spread
over the pillow at night. This permits a full circulation of
air to all the hair.

THE CARE OF YOUR BABY

REPRINT No. 727
from the
PUBLIC HEALTH REPORTS
February 3, 1922
WITH ADDITIONS AND DEDUCTIONS
by
DR. ST. LOUIS ESTES

Motherhood

Each year nearly a quarter of a million babies die in the United States. Of these, a large number could have been saved.

One hundred thousand of these babies die in the first month of life, most of them because of conditions affecting the mother before the baby was born. By giving proper care and attention to mothers before the baby is born, thousands of baby lives can be saved.

Thousands of mothers lose their lives needlessly. But mothers should have better care, for another important reason. In this country at least 15,000 mothers die in childbirth each year; that is, one mother in every 150 cases

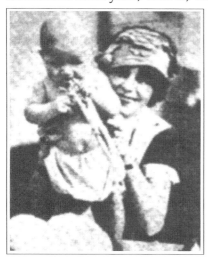

of childbirth. Over half of them lose their lives from preventable conditions. What can we do to stop this awful sacrifice?

Safeguarding the health of expectant mothers. In looking forward to the

With Dixie Lou Medora, at Five Months, Having her Raw Food Lunchs

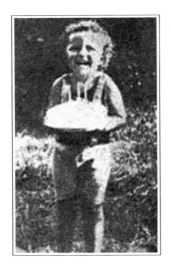

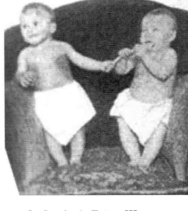

*Sr. Louis A. Estes, III
and Dixie Lou Medora Estes,
at 61/2 months.
The first Raw Food Twins.*

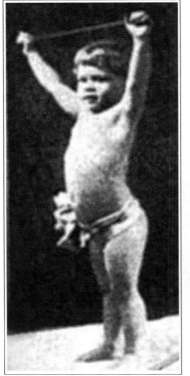

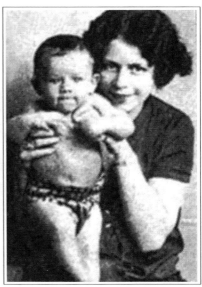

coming of her baby, the expectant mother should see that her home conditions are as favorable to her physical condition as it is possible to make them. She should not upset all her family affairs, but should so arrange them as to permit her to observe the following precautions:

Examination: Every expectant mother should early place herself under the care of a good physician who uses Natural Methods or a well-conducted maternity clinic or health center and have a complete physical examination made once in the early months of pregnancy and again during the last month, in order to know that all is well with her and with her child. If the expected baby is her first, the physical examination which the doctor makes should include measurements of the pelvis in order to determine if she may safely give birth to a child.

An examination of the blood by means of the Wassermann test shows that a certain percentage of expectant mothers should undergo thorough Nature treatment in order to insure a healthy baby.

Repeated examinations of the urine are essential for the detection of disease conditions the early discovery of which may save the mother's life. She should have her urine examined once every month up to the sixth month, and after that every ten days or two weeks. She should void at least three pints of urine every twenty-four hours.

Diet: Her food should be plain, wholesome and nutritious. She can eat anything that agrees with her in Raw Food. If she wishes to protect her health, retain her youth, have an easy childbirth and produce a strong, healthy baby, she should eliminate salt and live as much on Raw Foods, grains, cereals, nuts, buttermilk, fruit and fruit juices as possible. At least a quart of milk should be consumed daily. If you must have cooked food, confine it to soups and broths with very little seasoning. Chocolate, cocoa, tea, coffee, meat and salt should not be used at all, as they produce an excess acid condition and a stiffening and hardening of the nerve muscle tissue, causing the tissues of the uterus to become taut and lose their elasticity.

Fruits and vegetables keep the bowels open. Always eat lightly and more frequently. This system of eating is especially beneficial in morning sickness and vomiting.

Constipation. The bowels should move at least once every day. If constipation is troublesome, as it is likely to be in the later months of pregnancy, and does not readily respond to proper diet and exercise, these measures may be supplemented by the use of mineral oil or mild laxatives which should be prescribed by the physician.

Clothing. The clothing should be loose and comfortable, with no constricting bands or corsets. Special maternity corsets may be worn, and a corset cover with darts may be used to support the breasts. Shoes with low heels should be worn.

Exercise and fresh air. From one to two hours should be spent in the fresh air each day, preferably in walking or some other light form of exercise. Light housework is an excellent form of exercise. Expectant mothers should never be over-fatigued. Deep breathing should be practiced continuously off and on throughout the day. Ten deep breaths every two hours, always with light stretching exercises, drawing the muscles of the abdomen and groin out, like stretching a rubber band. By stretching the body out, thus stimulating the blood supply to these parts. If these parts are kept exercised childbirth will be much easier.

The patient should consume a glass of water for every fifteen pounds of her weight, keeping the body flushed from its excess poisons. It is well for her to lie down once or twice a day for a nap, with her feet elevated if there is a tendency for veins in the legs to enlarge. The last months of pregnancy she should avoid all heavy work, excessive use of the sewing machine and heavy lifting. This may bring on a miscarriage.

Sleeping. She should sleep at least eight hours every night, with the windows open. During the day the living rooms should be well ventilated.

Bathing. A warm bath at night, with soap, two or three times a week, and a cool morning bath and rubdown with a towel, will keep the skin in good condition and lighten the burden of the kidneys.   In bathing, avoid very hot or very cold water.

Dental Care. "A tooth for every child" no longer holds good. At the beginning of pregnancy she should consult a dentist and have her teeth put in good condition. Pregnancy is no longer considered a contra-indication to dental work. She should be sure to brush her teeth after each meal and rinse the mouth with limewater, which may be diluted with a little clear, cold water, if necessary. In fact, the most effective solvent to use as a mouth wash is limewater.

Miscarriages. If she has had one or more miscarriages or premature births, she should take a complete rest from two to three days each month at the time menstruation would have taken place were she not pregnant. The appearance of a bloody discharge demands instant summoning of the physician.

Care of the breasts. Few things can be done for the welfare of the baby which are so important as insuring the ability of the mother to nurse her baby. In the first year after birth, bottle-fed babies are four times more likely to die than are breast-fed babies. During the last two months of pregnancy the breasts should receive careful attention and treatment in preparation for nursing. The nipples should be anointed every night with white vaseline or albolene, which should be carefully removed in the morning with castile soap and warm water. If the nipples are small, flat or depressed, special treatment is needed and should be taken upon the advice of the physician.

Danger signals. If at any time during pregnancy she should suffer from severe and persistent vomiting, repeated or constant headache, dizziness, puffiness about the face, hands or legs, blurring of vision, spots before the eyes, scanty urine, muscular twitching, convulsions or bleeding, she should consult her physician without delay.

Preparation for confinement. She should not delay preparing the clothing for the expected baby. This may be done months ahead. Just before the expected date of confinement the room should be put in order and the material for preparing the bed for confinement should be kept readily at hand.

Patent medicines. A number of patent medicines have been widely advertised to make childbirth safe, easy and painless. They are all frauds. Instead of wasting money on them, expectant mothers should seek a doctor's advice.

The great event. At no time in her life does a woman require better care and attention than during childbirth. A competent doctor, or if such is not available, a properly supervised and licensed midwife, should attend. The patient's room should be large, clean and light, and the necessary maternity outfit should be conveniently at hand The following lists represent useful outfits:

LIST 1.
1   pound absorbent cotton
1   yard sterile gauze.
1   tube vaseline.
1   cake castile soap
1   flannel band, 5 inches wide,
1   yard long
6   bird's-eye diapers.
$\frac{1}{2}$ dozen small safety pins.
2   dozen large safety pins.
1   ounce powdered boracic acid.

LIST 2.

1 pound absorbent cotton.
5 yards sterile gauze.
1 envelope sterile umbilical tapes,
1 dozen sterile sanitary napkins.
1 tube vaseline.
4 ounces powdered boracic acid.
1 dozen bird's-eye diapers.
1 flannel band, 5 inches wide, 1 yard long.
1 cake, castile soap.
1 dozen small safety pins.
2 dozen large safety pins.
1 new douche bag, 2 quarts.
1 eye dropper.
1 douche pan.
$\frac{1}{2}$ yards rubber nursery sheeting.

After baby comes. The mother should rest in bed for two weeks after the baby is born and for several weeks more should not do really heavy work. Various forms of serious female troubles are due to a failure to follow this advice.

The mother's food should be plentiful, wholesome and nutritious; for, of course, baby must be nursed at the breast. The mother should drink plenty of milk, but tea and coffee are injurious.

Almost all mothers can breast-feed their babies.

If the flow of milk is scanty, the mother should—

(a) Drink plenty of barley and oatmeal water and fruit juices.
(b) Not do heavy work.
(c) Get sufficient rest and sleep.
(d) Take an outdoor airing every pleasant day.
(e) Avoid constipation.
(f) Put baby to nurse regularly.

In order to train the child and to keep herself well and strong, the mother should systematize baby's daily life, the nursing times, bath, sleep and outdoor periods. If the baby is often fretful, the mother should seek the doctor's advice. Under no circumstances should she give soothing syrups or other patent medicines recommended by the neighbors. *Register the baby's birth.* It is an important duty the mother owes her little one to make sure that his birth is properly recorded with the authorities. Ask the doctor if he registered your baby at the health department.

Here are some of the reasons why births should be recorded:

To establish identity and prove nationality.
To prove descent, or legitimacy.
To establish the right of inheritance to property.
To establish ability to make contracts.
To show when he has the right to enter school.
To show when he has the right to seek employment.
To establish the right to vote.
To establish the right to hold public office.
To enter the professions.
To prove the age at which the marriage contract may be entered into.
To establish liability to military duty.

For court purposes. Fill out this memorandum and preserve it for your baby. It may save him much time, money and inconvenience.

Baby a name _____

Date of birth: Day _____ Month _____ Year. _____

Sex _____

If twin or triplet, give number in order of birth _____

Birthplace _____ Birth registration No._____

Father' name _____ Birthplace _____

Mother's maiden name _____ Birthplace _____

Attending physician _____

Address _____

Baby's health history: There are many times when it is of the greatest importance to know something definite about the life history of a child. The following record is therefore suggested to all mothers. Keep this book handy and make your records in it. Use special memoranda pages in the back of the book for notes on your babies and children:

PERSONAL HISTORY

Date _____ Record made by _____

Weight at birth _____ pounds _____ Strong _____

Feeble _____ Premature _____

Birth registered _____ Registration No. _____

Number child of mother. 1, 2, 3, 4, 5, 6 , 7, 8, 9, 10, 11, 12 _____

Kind of food at present _____

Number feedings in 24 hours ____ Amount each feeding _____

Hours of feeding: Day _____ Night _____
Breast-fed from _____to _____ Weaned at what age _____

Bottle-fed from _____ to _____ What bottle food _____

Child sleeps alone _____ If not with whom _____

Awakenshour ____ Goes to bed ____hour ____ Sleeps well _____

Sleeps in open air. Day _____ Night _____
Sleeps with windows open _____

If table-fed, give chief articles of diet _____

Drinks tea _____ Coffee _____

Eats well _____ Eats good breakfast _____Bowels regular

ILLNESS
(Check each illness or condition separate and give age at attack)
CONTAGIONS

Measles _____ Whooping cough _____
Scarlet fever _____ Diphtheria _____ Chicken pox _____

Other _____

RESPIRATORY

Croup _____ Colds _____ Tonsillitis _____
Influenza or grippe _____ Bronchitis _____ Pneumonia _____
Other _____

DIGESTIVE

Constipation _____ Colic _____
Indigestion _____ Diarrhea _____
Other _____

OTHER ALIMENTS

Convulsions _____ Earache _____
Fevers _____ Enuresis (bed wetting) _____
Vaccination _____ Other inoculations _____

REMARKS

Bathing the Baby

Baby should be bathed at least once a day. During the hot weather one or two extra sponge baths may be given; but as a rule the daily bath should be a tub bath. A tub bath is preferable to the sponge bath for several reasons. It can be done more quickly and thoroughly, and the baby is not so liable to take cold.

The room should be warm; an open fire is desirable in cool weather. The water should be comfortably warm but not hot, about 90 to 95 deg. F. The temperature of the baby's bath may be tested with the bare elbow, never with the hand. However, a bath thermometer is the best method of testing the water. *Equipment.* Everything needed for the bath should be in readiness before baby is undressed. It is well to have a small wicker basket painted white, which will contain all the articles necessary for baby's toilet. In this should be kept a cake of pure white castile soap, a small bottle of olive oil, pure talcum powder, boric acid, four dozen safety pins of assorted sizes and a roll of absorbent cotton. Besides this, there should be in readiness a clean wash cloth, clean towels, full set of clean clothing.

Undressing. To undress the baby, take the clothes off over his feet. If held on the lap, a large bath towel should be placed across the lap to prevent his tender skin from coming in contact with the rough or worsted dress, and to receive him when he is lifted out of the tub. A more convenient way of bathing the baby is to undress him on a table instead of the lap. After undressing the baby, wrap him in a small blanket or large bath towel while washing his face.

Washing baby's face. Before putting the baby into the tub, wash his face, head and ears, being careful not to get soap into his eyes and mouth. Very little soap is needed for baby's skin. It is most important that the skin should be rinsed thoroughly. Pat the skin dry with a soft towel, taking care to dry well back of the ears and in the soft folds of the neck. The eyes should be cleansed with absorbent cotton dipped in boric acid solution. Squeeze a drop into each eye, being careful to use a fresh piece of cotton for each eye. The mouth and nose then should be cleansed with an applicator dipped in boric acid solution. An applicator is made by twisting a small tuft of absorbent cotton upon the end of a wooden toothpick in such a way as to make a rounded pad. If made correctly, the cotton will not slip off readily. Be careful not to injure the ears. It is better to ask your physician or the nurse to show you just how to cleanse the ears correctly.

The tub bath. It is well to lay a bath towel in the bottom of the tub and put only a small amount of water in at first, so as not to frighten the baby. If baby is plunged immediately into a tub of water, it becomes startled and may never enjoy a tub bath; whereas if the water is added gradually, the baby's attention in the meantime being attracted to something else, it soon learns to enjoy the morning dip.

Before placing baby into the tub, soap the entire body thoroughly; then place him in the bath, holding him with the left forearm under the neck and shoulders, the left hand under his arm, and lifting the feet and legs with right hand. Support the baby while in the tub with the left hand and arm. Sponge the entire body with the right hand; then lift the baby out and wrap him in a bath towel. Dry carefully with the soft towel, patting the skin gently. Never rub the baby's tender skin with anything less smooth than the palm of the hand. A little pure talcum powder may be used in the creases and folds of the skin, under the arms, and around the buttocks; but it should not be used so freely as to clog the pores of the skin, and never should be used until the skin has been dried as thoroughly as possible with the towel.

The baby's bath should be given as nearly as possible at the same hour each day, at least an hour after feeding. At first the duration of the bath should be only about three minutes. Later it may be five minutes, and as the child grows older and stronger he may be allowed to play in the water for about fifteen minutes, as the skin absorbs some water, which is beneficial to the system. Besides this, the water relaxes the muscles and aids in overcoming many wrong conditions. Muscles that have been contracted by disease will be benefited by the warm bath.

Bran baths. When there is any irritation of the skin, such as chafing or prickly heat, oatmeal bags or bran may be substituted for soap. Make a *cotton* bag of cheesecloth or other thin material and fill loosely with bran. Soak the bag in the bath water, squeezing it until it becomes milky.

Powder. A little pure talcum powder may be used in the creases and folds of the skin, under the arms, and around the buttocks; but it should not be used too freely, for reasons already mentioned. A highly-perfumed powder should not be used.

An older child who does not want to take a bath may be taught to enjoy it by having some toy added to the bath, such as one of the floating animals that may be purchased for as little as five cents apiece. It is much better to coax a child with some toy than to compel him by force against his will. In training a child, one never should attempt to "break" his will, but rather should endeavor to guide it in right channels. Strong-willed (not stubborn) people make the best citizens. Many a child has been made stubborn by attempts to coerce him into submission.

Caution

Babies are left to lie in their soiled napkins very frequently by a careless and too-often busy mother. The excreta and urine have an irritating effect upon the tender and delicate flesh of the baby, so that after careless washing the baby will go into a crying spell and become fussy and irritable. These conditions not only ruin the disposition of the baby, but frequently lead to doping in the effort of the mother to ascertain the trouble and quiet the baby. So many mothers in their hurry remove soiled diapers (especially when the baby has only urinated) and hurriedly wipe the baby with a wet cloth, dry quickly and powder. The urine on the little body has become partly soaked into the pores of the skin. I want to caution against these rush bathings. If you do not want to ruin the disposition and produce irritation and crying spells that you cannot understand, be sure to bathe the parts with warm water thoroughly, to remove all the urine. Look for the trouble here when it cannot be located elsewhere.

Development of the Baby

At birth a baby's head is larger in proportion to his body than is an adult's. The abdomen is big. The arms and legs are short, and the legs are slightly bowed.

Soon after birth a baby develops sense of contact and temperature—that is, he knows when he is being held and he can appreciate heat or cold. He learns to see light and to hear during the first three or four days.

The first month the hands move aimlessly about. During the second month he learns to put his hand to his mouth and tries to lift his head.

During the third and fourth months a baby will make an effort to grasp what is held before him and will try to sit up. He should not be allowed to do so unless he is supported. About this time he begins to recognize others and develops a will of his own, which is expressed in crying when he is displeased. He will coo when he is happy.

About the sixth month a baby can sit alone for a few minutes. He will grasp and hold whatever comes within reach of his busy fingers. He now begins to be sociable and will try to talk, sometimes making vowel sounds.

From the seventh month to the ninth month he will creep and will make efforts to stand. He likes to imitate movements and to have sympathy and attention shown him.

From the ninth month to the twelfth month he learns to stand, and from the twelfth to the sixteenth month learns to walk. He develops a sense of desire to please, and this leads to obedience. Sometimes at the twelfth month he can say a few words.

A baby simply follows his instincts. An older person must keep him from harm and show him gently how to do the right things until he learns for himself.

Weigh your baby. The loss of a pound or two of weight makes very little difference to the adult, but it is a serious matter for a young baby. A pound or two loss means as much to the baby as ten or fifteen pounds does to the adult, for it is 10 per cent or more of his total body weight.

If a baby fails to gain in weight for several weeks, or loses a pound or two, it becomes noticeable. But the average daily gain in weight for the first year is so small that it cannot be detected without weighing.

It is very much easier to keep a young baby well and gaining steadily than it is to have him regain lost weight, or to get him well again once he has become ill. For these reasons a mother should weigh the young baby every week until he is nine months old, and after that at least every two weeks until he is one year old. From infancy until he enters school the child should be weighed at least once a month.

The average baby weighs a little over seven pounds at birth. He doubles his weight at six months, weighing ordinarily fourteen pounds, and triples it at one year, weighing about twenty-one pounds.

Get to Know Your Baby

Babies cannot talk, but they have a sign language which the observant mother may learn to understand. By proper interpretation of his crying and movements, a great many of baby's wants may be determined and wisely cared for.

What to observe in a baby: A normal, healthy child gains regularly in weight, has a warm, moist skin, breathes quietly, eats heartily, sleeps peacefully, has one or two regular bowel movements daily, and cries only when he is hungry, uncomfortable, ill, or indulging in a fit of temper.

Posture when sleeping: Quiet, limbs relaxed, sleep peaceful, no tossing about.

Facial expression: Calm and peaceful. If baby is suffering pain, the features will contract from time to time, and the fists will be clenched tightly.

Breathing: Regular, easy, and quiet; however, during the first weeks of life breathing may be irregular in perfectly normal babies. This should excite no alarm unless associated with other abnormal conditions, such as hot skin and flushed face.

Baby should breathe through the nose and keep the mouth closed. Mouth breathing or habitual holding the mouth open usually indicates enlarged tonsils or adenoids or some other obstruction to the breathing which needs the attention of a physician.

Skin: Warm, slightly moist, and a healthy pink color. The skin should be soft and smooth to the touch, and the underlying muscles firm. Flabby muscles usually indicate something wrong with the feeding.

Crying: Babies need a certain amount of crying to develop their lungs. When children cry for everything they want, it is the result of faulty training. If baby is cross or fretful and cries a great deal of time it does not mean necessarily that he is ill, but there is something wrong with him. Learn what he is trying to tell you by crying.

Hunger Cry: A low whimpering cry sometimes accompanied by sucking the fingers or the lips. If the meal is not forthcoming, it may change to a lusty scream. Babies are as likely to cry from indigestion caused by overfeeding as from hunger.

Fretful Crying: The baby is sleepy or uncomfortable. He may be too warm or tired of being laid in one position. A tepid sponge bath and gentle rub or a change of clothing and taking him out will prove very restful and comforting. If the crying continues, consult the doctor; the child may be ill.

Cry of Colic or Pain: A lusty cry sometimes rising to a shriek, with tears in the eyes. In colic or abdominal pain the knees are drawn up and the fists are clenched. A tight fist is usually an indication of pain. If the crying increases, with moving of an arm or leg or when placing the child in a certain position, he may have a broken bone or other damage calling for the attention of a doctor.

Sick Cry: The very sick baby does not cry hard. There is low moaning or a wail, with sometimes a turning of the head from side to side.

Sick Baby. Learn to recognize any change from the normal. Unusual flushing or pallor of the face, sleeplessness, lack of energy, loss of appetite, profuse sweating, especially of the head, peevishness, vomiting or diarrhea, give warning that something is wrong. Find out what and why.

How to handle a baby: A baby must always be handled carefully. His bones are still part cartilage, and they bend and break easily. Other bad effects of too much or careless handling are sore and painful muscles, which make a baby cross. Handling after eating upsets the digestion. Jolting, bouncing and rocking make a child excitable and nervous.

A young baby cannot turn himself over, and his muscles get very tired if he remains too long in one position. When he is taken up for feeding or cleansing, his position should be changed from side to side, or from lying on his back. But always the head and back must be kept straight and the arms and legs free. The ears should be kept straight and flat on the head. The eyes should be protected from direct light.

To hold a young baby on one arm, lay him flat on his back on your left arm, supporting the neck and head with the palm of the hand and fingers, and pressing his body close to your body with the left elbow.   Never throw a baby over the shoulder.

A baby should not be encouraged to try to hold up his own head until he is four months old or to sit up until he is six months old. The spine, back and head always should be supported. Never pick a child up by the arms. Grasp him firmly by the shoulders or body.

In walking with an older child do not walk too fast nor compel him to reach up to take your hand. It is very tiring to walk in that position.

Baby's daily program: A baby must have regular hours for nursing and for sleep. He must be put to bed on time at the same time every day.

The baby's bath, outing, play time, nap, going to stool, in fact everything that is necessary to a baby's care, should be done with the same care, precision and regularity that is used in caring for any fine machine.

Regularity in baby's care will establish good habits. The first years of a child's life are, for these reasons, the most important. If he has the right sort of care then, and is trained in the right sort of habits from the very first day of his life, he will grow and develop properly.

On the other hand, careless and irregular feeding, keeping baby awake at all hours, waking him to show to the neighbors, taking him out to walk when he ought to be in bed, will make a baby unhappy and cross.

A child who has been trained to habits of regularity, to obedience and self-control, is much more easily taken care of when ill and these habits assist in the recovery.

Sample Program for Every Day

6 A. M.—Baby's first nursing.
Family breakfast; children off to school.
9 A. M.—Baby's bath, followed by second nursing.
Baby sleeps until noon.
12.—Baby's noon meal.
Out-of-door airing and nap.
3 P. M.—Afternoon nursing.
Period of waking.
6 P. M.—Baby's supper and bed.
10to 12 P. M.—Baby's night meal.

Breast-Feeding the Baby

The most loving act a mother can do is nurse her baby. When nursing, it not only gets the best food, but it is less liable to many diseases, such as summer complaint, convulsions and tuberculosis.

Of every 100 breast-fed babies, 6 die in the first year of life; whereas of every 100 bottle-fed babies, 25 die in the first year of life. The baby will have the best chance of living if he is fed at the breast.

A baby should be breast-fed exclusively except when the supply of breast milk is insufficient to make him gain properly. Nearly every mother can nurse her baby during the first three or four months of life; and if she can nurse it for 10 months, so much the better.

Even if there is but little breast milk at first, there may be an abundant supply after the first few weeks. The act of nursing causes the milk to come into the breast and increase the supply.

Maintenance of breast feeding: Mothers who previously have experienced difficulty in nursing, and those who are anxious regarding the ability to continue nursing, should realize that the quickest way to dry up the breasts is to omit one or more nursing's, under the mistaken impression that by so doing they are saving up the milk.

If a mother is not utilizing her full milk supply, from inability of the infant to nurse properly, from the necessity of temporarily discontinuing nursing, or from other causes, she can preserve the ability to breast-feed by thoroughly emptying the breasts after each feeding, or at regular nursing intervals, by manual expression. This is accomplished by placing the thumb and forefinger of one hand from one-half inch to one inch beyond the colored areola surrounding the nipple, and with a "back-down-out" motion, as in milking, express the milk. Mothers readily acquire facility in emptying the breasts by this method, which is much more satisfactory than the use of the breast pump.

The mother's health: The nursing mother needs plenty of fresh air and some exercise each day in the open air, preferably walking or light gardening. The ordinary household duties may be performed but the nursing mother must not be overworked. She should take a nap each afternoon, or at least lie down and rest in a cool room.

The nursing mother cannot afford to have a spell of nerves. Anger, worry, grief, excitement all interfere with the nervous system and its control of the circulation of the blood, which affects the supply and the quality of the milk.

Rules for nursing: The mother should lie down to nurse her baby. The newborn baby is put to the breast when he is 5 or 6 hours old. During the first 24 hours he should nurse not more than four times, but at both breasts each time. A newborn baby may be given plain, cool, boiled water at regular intervals between nursing. Do not give him any kind of tea or other mixture.

Beginning with the second day, baby should nurse every two and one-half to three hours. On the three-hour schedule he nurses at 6, 9, and 12 noon etc until 4 months old.   Alternate each breast or let him take both breasts at each time, according to his appetite and the amount of milk. In the event the milk is delayed longer than the third day, baby should be fed from the bottle at three-hour intervals; but he should be put to the breast regularly in order to stimulate the flow of milk.

The average healthy baby nurses every three hours until it is 4 months old. When he is 6 months old, he nurses every four hours, usually taking both breasts each time. This makes six nursing's in 24 hours, four during the day and one at night, as follows: 6 A. M., 10 A. M., 2 P. M., 6 P. M., 10 P. M, and at 2 A. M.

Convenient hours for nursing.

(1)   Eight nursing's in 24 hours: 6 A. M., 9 A. M., 12 noon, 3 P. M., 6 P. M., 9 P. M., 12 midnight, and once during the night.

(2)   Six nursing's in 24 hours: 6 A. M., 9 A. M., 12 noon, 2 P. M., 6 P. M., and at the mother's bedtime; or at 6 A. M., 10 A. M., 2 P. M., 6 P. M., 10 P. M., and once during the night.

(3)   Five nursing's in 24 hours: Six A. M., 10 A. M., 2 P. M., 6 P. M., 10 P. ML, or later.

Regularity. It is very important to follow regular hours for nursing. If baby is fed every time he cries, his digestion soon will be upset. If he cries between feedings, give him plain cooled boiled water. Babies are as likely to cry from overfeeding as from hunger.

Length of time of nursing. The length of time of nursing varies with the infant and with the breast. The average infant rarely nurses longer than fifteen minutes. The important point is to satisfy the baby. If there is any doubt, let the baby nurse longer, but not more than twenty minutes. If it is not satisfied after 20 minutes, consult a physician.

Water for the baby. The baby should be offered cooled, boiled water between feedings. Beginning with a teaspoonful during the first few days after birth, the quantity of water should be gradually increased until the baby is taking from five to six ounces of water daily.

Boil a pint of fresh water every morning, put it in a clean bottle, and keep in a cool place. Do not give the baby ice water.

Orange juice. The baby should be given fresh orange juice each day, preferably just before his second nursing. Beginning with one teaspoonful when the baby is one month old, the amount should be gradually increased, until by the time he is a year old he is taking from one to three tablespoonfuls. Strained tomato juice may be given in like proportion when oranges are not available. Also prune juice.

Weaning. A baby should not be fed at the breast after the age of one year. At that age he needs a more solid food to make him grow strong.

A baby should be weaned gradually, and the milk at first should be only half the strength of the formula used for a normal child of the same age. Then the milk should be gradually increased in strength.

Weaning may usually begin at about the ninth month, by giving baby one feeding of cow's milk, using two parts of milk to one part water, and if he digests this well the amount of water can be decreased gradually until at ten or eleven months he may be taking the whole milk. And remember, all milk feedings can be slowly increased as the breast feedings are decreased, until at one year of age the baby is weaned entirely. A baby weaned at nine or ten months may be taught to take milk from a cup. At about the eighth or ninth month the baby should be given the juices from beets, carrots, turnips, lettuce leaves and from all vegetables from which juices can be extracted—using the juices for this purpose.

A liquid broth may be made from ground whole cereal, such as whole wheat, barley, rye, corn and oats. Grind cereal fine or soak overnight in fresh water and strain. Thicken it, when preparing, with milk.

Train the baby to take its food in the natural state and abstain from sweetening the prepared foods. Do not cultivate an artificial taste for sugars and sweets. Preserve the health of your child in its infancy. It should also be given nut milk, prepared by grinding the nuts to a fine powder and pressing them.

A baby one year of age in July should not be weaned during the hot months if he is doing well. It is dangerous to wean a young baby. It should not be done for the convenience of the mother and should never be done without the advice of a physician. Infants should be weaned where the mothers are suffering from a disease which they might transmit to the child—such as typhoid fever or—tuberculosis—and if the mother is suffering from some disease which might be aggravated by nursing, such as Bright's disease, tuberculosis or acute pneumonia. The infant should likewise be weaned if the mother becomes pregnant or if she is suffering from inflammation of the breasts.

Mixed feeding: When the mother's milk is diminishing, it is advisable to make up the lack with prepared modified cows milk. This may be done either by following one or more breast feedings with enough modified milk to satisfy the baby or by giving one or more full bottle feedings instead of the like number of breast feedings The flow of breast milk tends to diminish when the baby nurses less than five times in twenty-four hours. When the baby is being nursed every four hours and is not satisfied, it is better to give him, after nursing, enough modified milk to satisfy him rather than to replace a nursing with a bottle. If, on the other hand, shorter intervals and more feedings are being used, a bottle feeding may take the place of the nursing without so much danger of decreasing the supply of breast milk. Most babies need additional food after the seventh month.

Follow the raw food recipes in this book and you will not have to worry about the quality or the amount of your milk supply. Living on the raw foods prior to childbirth will save many a woman from being torn and the conditions that produce invalids throughout life and necessitate operations.

Thyroid gland. Remember that cooked food produces the poisons that cause children's diseases. The thyroid gland regulates the growth and health by controlling the elimination of albuminous poisons in the bowels. This gland does not commence to develop until about three years of age. This is one of the reasons why children should not be fed anything containing beef broth or have meat of any kind.

The lack of calcium in the meat prevents the proper development of the bones of the child. The acids produced by the action of the meat and the cooked foods deprive the muscles and nerves of their strength and produce acidosis of the tissues. The child has no protection against its childish diseases, such as anemia, nervousness, catarrh, polypus, adenoids, scarlet fever, measles, mumps, rickets, infantile paralysis, Saint Vititus' dance and spinal meningitis, because of the fact the poisons are not being eliminated by the action of the thyroid gland. The only remedy, therefore, is nature's remedy of Raw Foods, which carry all the minerals necessary to absorb the acid poisons of the body and too build strong nerve muscle and bone tissue also sweeping the bowels and overcoming the bacterial condition there.

If you eat nature's foods in their natural state you will not need to worry about the health and strength of your child or the ordinary diseases that they are commonly afflicted with.

Bottle feeding for babies: When the doctor decides that breast feeding cannot be carried out, cow's milk is the most satisfactory substitute for mother's milk. The best milk (this does not mean the richest milk) is none too good. Get certified milk, if possible. If you cannot obtain certified milk, get the cleanest and purest bottled milk you can find, preferably pasteurized milk. Milk sold in bulk, or bottled from the can in stores or by milkmen in their wagons, is likely to be stale and contaminated and not a proper food for the baby, even though it looks and tastes good. "Baby foods" and condensed milks and the like are not satisfactory substitutes for good cow's milk, and are not good for prolonged feeding

Equipment. Select good quality of granite ware for the utensils for preparing baby's milk, and never use them for any other purpose. They must always be kept scrupulously clean and scalded each time before using. The following are essential:

  1 large pan with inverted pie pan in the bottom for pasteurizing,
  1 two-quart granite saucepan, with handle, or pitcher,
  1 table spoon,
  1 pint measure,
  7 bottles; corks and nipples for each bottle,
  1 wire rack for holding bottles,
  1 bottle brush,
  1 fruit jar for cereal water,
  1 box of baking soda or borax.

Bottles: Select bottles with smooth, round sides and marked for the different quantities of food. There should be as many bottles as there are feedings in twenty-four hours. The bottle should be cleaned immediately after feeding by rinsing in clear water, then by soaking in suds, borax or soap water. Bottles should be scrubbed with a clean brush in warm soapsuds and rinsed *with boiling water.* (Then they should be filled with boiled water until ready for use.) The corks should be scalded each day and kept in a tightly-cove red receptacle.

Nipples: Use only non-collapsible nipples that can be slipped over the neck of the bottle.

After each feeding cleanse the nipple inside and outside, scrubbing it with a brush in warm soapy water. Wrap the nipples in a clean cloth and boil them once a day. Drop them into a scalded jelly glass and put the lid on tight. Never touch with your fingers that part of the nipple which must go into the baby's mouth. The hole in the nipple should be only large enough to allow the drops to fall about one and one-half inches apart when the bottle is inverted.

How to feed baby: Babies that are artificially fed should be under the supervision of a physician, who should see them at regular intervals. Very young babies, or those that are not thriving, should always be seen once a week, and older, healthy babies should be seen at least once a month, whether they are sick or well. The following rules and suggestions apply to all bottle-fed babies:

Feed the baby by the clock: When it is feeding time, shake the bottle gently to mix the contents and place it in a pan of hot water to warm it. Test the temperature by letting a few drops fall on the inside of the wrist.

Giving the bottle: The bottle should always be held while the child is taking the food. The baby should be lying down while feeding. Do not allow him to drink longer than twenty minutes. Do not urge him to take more than he wants. If he does not take the whole feeding, throw out that remaining in the bottle; do not save it for another time.

A child should not be played with after feeding. He should not be allowed to suck on an empty bottle nor allowed to sleep or play with the nipple in his mouth.

After feeding, the child should be placed upright and patted gently to allow him to bring up gas or air which he has swallowed. He should then be placed in the bed, but not rocked.

Patent foods: There are many patent foods offered for sale, but as a rule they are expensive and have a tendency to make fat babies rather than strong babies. While they may be used for a short time, no baby should be fed on them exclusively.

Condensed milk: Condensed milk is not the same as fresh milk, and its continued use for a baby is likely to cause indigestion and a disease known as rickets. It is lacking in some of the necessary food elements and is therefore undesirable as a permanent food for children. Condensed milk is not cheaper than fresh cow's milk, although it may appear to cost less.

Powdered milk: When fresh cow's milk cannot be obtained, or when it is necessary to travel with the baby, powdered milk (whole milk containing three and one-half per cent butter fat) may be used as a substitute.

Important advice. When the baby has diarrhea, either with or without vomiting, stop all food at once and send for a physician immediately. Meantime allow baby to have plenty of boiled water to drink. Save the soiled diapers for the physician to examine. (Always keep them covered.) Give no medicine without the doctor's advice.

If the baby refuses to drink unsweetened, cooled, boiled water, give it barley or oatmeal water.

Be sure to wash the hands thoroughly after changing a diaper and before preparing food. Boil all the soiled diapers for fifteen minutes to kill the dangerous germs which might spread the diarrhea among the other members of the household.

If baby does not gain regularly in weight, or if he frets and cries a great deal, take him to the doctor and follow the doctor's advice.

Modification of Milk: The best known substitute for mother's milk is properly modified cow's milk. Pure, fresh, cow's milk contains all the food elements necessary for the growth and development of the baby.

A young baby cannot readily digest plain cow's milk, and so the milk must be modified according to the age and size of the baby and its powers of digestion. "Modified milk" is milk to which water or other substances have been added so as to make it suitable for a baby's stomach.

Ordinarily the milk may be increased by one-half ounce every eight days. The water may be decreased by one-half ounce every eight days.

If your baby does not gain properly and remain well, take it to your doctor, who may make the necessary change.

A newborn baby needs very little food for the first day or two. The first feeding should be made of one ounce of milk to two or three ounces of water. No food or substance other than cool, boiled water should be given except by the direction of the physician.

Regular increase in weight, as determined by the weekly weightings, is the indication that baby's food is not only agreeing with him and satisfying his hunger, but that it is also meeting his growth requirements.

Preparation: Sample formula for a six-month-old baby: Milk—26 ounces. Water—14 ounces.

Five feedings during the day, at four-hour intervals. Pasteurize in bottles.

Wash hands clean with soap, water and brush.

Scald utensils and place them conveniently on the table.

Wipe the top of the milk bottle with damp cloth to remove particles of dust.

Invert bottles several times to mix cream. Use nursing bottle or graduated measure to measure quantities; mix the materials thoroughly in a pitcher or pan.

Pour seven ounces of the mixture into each of the five bottles and lightly close the bottles with a plug of absorbent cotton.

Place bottles on inverted pan in kettle of water and pasteurize.

Cool bottles rapidly and put on ice.

Milk should be Pasteurized: Raw milk may carry the germs of tuberculosis, scarlet fever, tonsillitis, diphtheria, typhoid fever and other communicable diseases. Unless certified milk is used, this danger should be prevented by buying pasteurized milk or by pasteurizing or scalding the milk at home.

Pasteurization means heating the milk to about 150 deg. F. for thirty minutes and then rapidly cooling it. Milk for the baby should always be pasteurized in the feeding bottle. It may be done as follows: The milk should be mixed and poured into the clean feeding bottles, which should then be stopped with clean, non-absorbent cotton. It is then ready for pasteurization. While a number of satisfactory pasteurizers may be bought in the shops, a homemade pasteurizer can be easily constructed.

Take a wire basket that will hold the six or seven bottles used in twenty-four hours' feeding, and place this basket containing the bottles in a tin bucket of cold water filled to a point a little above the level of the milk. Heat the water and allow it to boil for five minutes. Then set it to one side for ten minutes more, after which run cold water into the bucket until the milk is cooled to the temperature of the running water. The milk is then put into the ice chest, which should not be warmer than 50 deg. F.

If the baby's milk is to be mixed with other ingredients, such as oatmeal, barley water, rice water, etc., these should be added to the milk before pasteurization. When the milk is once prepared, the bottle should not be opened until it is given to the baby.

Milk should be kept cold: After the baby's milk has been prepared, it is very important that it should be kept cold until it is used.

A simple icebox can be made as follows:

Get a wooden box at a grocery store, such as a soap box, fifteen inches in depth. Buy a covered earthenware crock, tall enough to hold a quart bottle of milk, also get a piece of oilcloth or linoleum about one foot wide and three feet long. Sew the ends together to make a cylinder which will fit loosely around the crock. Place the crock inside the oilcloth cylinder, and stand them in the center of the box. Now pack sawdust or excelsior beneath and all about them to keep the heat from getting in. Complete the refrigerator by nailing a Sunday paper or two other newspapers to the wooden cover of the box.

How to use the refrigerator. In the morning as soon as you receive the milk place it in the crock crack 5 cents' worth of ice and place it about the milk bottle. Place the cover on the crock and the lid on the wooden box. No matter how hot the day has been, you will find some unmelted ice in the crock the next morning. Remove the crock every morning to pour off the melted ice.

Orange juice: Not later than one month after being put on the bottle, or at any time from three months of age up, the infant should be given orange juice, beginning with one teaspoonful mixed with equal quantity of cooled boiled water and gradually increasing the quantity to two to three tablespoonfuls. The best time to give orange juice is just before the bath in the morning. Strained tomato juice may be given in like proportion when oranges are not available. The use of these juices will prevent scurvy.

Feeding the Baby After the First Year

The change from bottle or breast to table food must be made intelligently if the baby is to continue to grow properly. The same care must be exercised with regard to the regularity of meals and the character and the amount of food as with younger babies. The tendency is to overfeed babies of this age, especially by giving too much fat. A baby should not be given cream, and it may be necessary to remove a part of the cream when the milk is very rich. Too much fat in the food causes the formation of gas in the bowels, white stools, loss of appetite and pallor.

To try to feed a young baby at the family table while attempting to partake of a meal is not conducive to a mother's or father's digestion. It is also unfair to a young child to expect him to sit quietly through the time his elders take for their meal and not want the food he sees them eating.

A simple, safe and satisfactory method of feeding a young child, and a practical substitute for the always dangerous high chair is the separate small table and chair. Where the houseroom space is limited, this small table may be fastened on hinges to the wall so that it may be dropped out of the way when not in use.

While the mother is preparing the family meal, the baby may be served just what he ought to have at his own table. In this way he does not see other foods and will not ask for them. When baby has finished his own meal he will be content to play or sleep while the family enjoys theirs unhampered by his presence.

The small table is an excellent means of training in table manners. When the child has learned proper control of himself at the age of four or five years, the family will then enjoy his presence at their table.

Vitamins: It is now known that a diet composed only of meat, potatoes, bread and cereals does not promote the best growth and development of children. Such a diet should be supplemented by an abundance of milk, butter and the green, leafy vegetables, such as spinach, kale, lettuce, Swiss chard, onions, cress and beet and turnip tops. These articles of food are rich in the growth-stimulating "vitamins." Growing children should partake of them freely.

The diet of the child must be arranged with regard to his age and his ability to digest certain articles of food.

The Baby's Sleep, Rest and Play:

Baby's room. If the house is small, it is better to do without a parlor, which is not often used, and give one room to the little folks who will use it every day.

Sunshine is as necessary for babies as for plants. A baby not given sunshine will droop and pine just as the plant does. Therefore, choose a sunny room for the baby's room and one which has windows and doors on opposite sides so that a continual abundant supply of fresh air may be obtained.

The baby's room should be kept comfortably warm in winter. Furnace heat is better than stoves. Oil and gas stoves exhaust the air in a short time. An open grate is a great convenience both for the additional heat and because it helps to keep the air of the room in circulation. The floor should be bare, so that it can be kept clean by wiping it with a damp cloth or dust mop. A few washable rugs may be added. Plain white sash curtains should be provided at the windows, as they can be laundered frequently.

Fresh air. Fresh air is essential for the healthy baby. To obtain the best air without drafts, put baby's bed in the middle of the room. The windows may be opened from the top. They should be screened against flies and disease-carrying insects. Windows facing the hot sun should be provided with awnings. In the wintertime, a plentiful supply of fresh air without drafts may be obtained by tacking thin muslin or cheesecloth over the open windows or on the window screen. This also keeps out particles of coal, soot, dirt, and snow.

All the furnishings for the baby's room should be of the simplest kind, and such as can be wiped readily with a damp cloth or laundered and so kept free from dust. The equipment may include a screen to protect baby from drafts, a low chair without arms for the mother, baby scales, bathtub, basket for toilet articles, and plain table. A chest of drawers or bureau is a welcome convenience.

Bed: Baby's first bed may be made in an ordinary clothes basket, lined with a sheet. This can be picked up and carried about easily, which is an advantage. It should be placed on a chair or a box, never on the floor.

A feather pillow is not suitable for a mattress or for the baby's head. Use an old, soft comforter or ordinary mattress of hair, felt, or cotton, protected by rubber sheeting, light oilcloth, or paper blanket. Since rubber or oilcloth is hard and uncomfortable, a soft washable pad should be used directly underneath the sheet. Table felting makes an excellent pad for this purpose.

The young baby will breathe more easily and take a larger supply of air into his lungs if no pillow is used. A clean, soft folded napkin may be placed under his head.

Toward the end of the second year a thin hair pillow may be used.

Sleep: The child's body develops faster during the first year of his life than at any other period. For that reason a baby needs a large allowance of sleep, with the best sleeping accommodations, so that the hours of sleep may be of the greatest value to him.

Baby should sleep alone. Babies may be smothered to death while in bed with an older person, some part of whose body may be thrown over baby's face while asleep.

Medical authorities agree that babies need the following amount of sleep:

Age	Hour of sleep
Up to one month	18 to 20
One month to one year	16
One to two year	12

A baby should have the longest period of unbroken sleep at night and should not be permitted to turn night into day. Babies grow mainly while sleeping, and a fretful baby is a tired baby that has not had sufficient sleep.

The baby should be nursed at 6 P. M. and put to bed for the night in a quiet room. He is nursed again when the mother retires, between 10 and 12 P. M, and, when properly trained, will sleep until time for his first morning nursing at 6 A. M. Babies are easily trained to sleep the night through, thus allowing the mother to have an undisturbed night's rest so essential for her well-being, and that of the baby.

Daytime sleep: The daytime naps should be continued through the sixth year. The baby should never take a nap in all his clothes. The shoes of older children, especially, should be removed. In hot weather, remove all but the shirt and diaper from the baby.

The sleeping room should be darkened and well ventilated. The baby should be fed and made comfortable in every way, put in his crib, and let alone to go to sleep. He should never be rocked to sleep nor jolted nor bounced.

Sleeping out of doors: Out-of-door sleeping in summer, both by day and by night, is good for the baby after he is a month old. He must be protected from flies and mosquitoes, shielded from the wind and sun, and covered, if there is a sudden drop in temperature. The sleeping porch must be protected properly by canvas curtains, and in cold weather a hot-water bottle should be placed in baby's bed.

The baby must have an abundant supply of fresh air day and night. He should be kept out of doors as much as possible, avoiding the hot sun and also days when the thermometer drops below 22 deg. F., because of the danger of the face being frostbitten. In the summer time a newborn baby may be taken out of doors the first week. Begin with a daily outing of fifteen minutes about noon and gradually lengthen the time in the forenoon and afternoon until the baby is out from 10 o'clock until 2 o'clock. He must be clothed properly according to the weather, and his eyes must be protected from the sun. The baby carriage must be one in which the child can lie comfortably at full length and stretch his arms and legs. When sitting up, his little spine and feet must be supported properly.

Rest and Play

Rest: A young baby needs rest and quiet. However strong he may be, too much playing is bad, and it is likely to result in a restless night.

Rocking the baby, jumping him up and down on the knees, tossing him in constant motion, is very bad for him. These things disturb the baby's nerves and make him more and more dependent upon these attentions. When the young baby is awake he should be taken up frequently and held quietly in the arms in various positions, so that no one set of muscles may become tired. An older child should be taught to sit on the floor or in his pen or crib and amuse himself during the part of his waking hours. Baby must never be lifted by the arms.

Toys: Since a baby wants to put everything in his mouth, his toys must be those that can be used safely in this way. They should be washable and should have no sharp points or corners to hurt the eyes. Painted articles, or hairy and woolly toys, also toys having loose parts, such as balls or objects small enough to be swallowed, are unsafe and should never be given a small child.

A baby should never have too many toys at one time. A handful of clothespins or a silver teaspoon or tin cup will please just as much as an expensive doll or other toy. It is a good plan to have a box or basket in which to keep empty spools and other household objects with which the baby may play.

The Baby's Clothing

In dressing the baby, he should be handled as little as possible. A little baby's body is very tender, and if handled roughly or too much he will be made very uncomfortable. All the clothing should be drawn on and off over the feet instead of over the head.

When he is dressed completely, baby has on a band, shirt, diaper, skirt, dress, and bootees. None of this clothing should be heavy or stiff. It is better to dress a baby lightly and slip on a little short jacket for cool mornings and evenings. When baby is a few months old, it is a good plan on a hot summer day to take off all his clot thing for a few minutes in the middle of the day and allow him to roll and play on a bed.

Elaborate or fancy trimmed garments have no place in a little baby's wardrobe. Both mother and baby are better off without them, especially if the mother must care for the garments herself. Starched garments, and lace about the neck of a little baby's dress, are liable to irritate the tender skin and cause the child a great deal of discomfort. Sometimes these irritations are difficult to heal.

For the first few weeks of life the new baby does little but eat, sleep, and grow. He needs many clean clothes, and these should be of the simplest and most comfortable kind.

The following are all that are necessary:

Band: Three flannel abdominal bands made of soft, white, un-hemmed flannel, five or six inches wide and from fourteen to eighteen inches long. They should be wide enough to protect the abdomen and not wide enough to wrinkle. They should go once and a half around the baby's abdomen, lap across the front, and pin at the side. After the cord is healed, these may be replaced by three knitted abdominal bands with shoulder straps and a tab to pin to the diaper. The lower part of these should be made of wool and the upper part of cotton. This kind of band will not slip around the baby's chest and make him uncomfortable. The band may be discarded altogether in hot weather.

Shirts: Three shirts, wool and cotton, or wool and silk, never all wool. For the very hottest weather, an all cotton or silk shirt may be worn. The shirts should be fitted smoothly. They may either lap or button in front.

Stockings: Three pairs of bootees; three pairs of merino or cashmere stockings if the weather is cold.

Blankets: Three blankets of closely-knitted or crocheted wool, or made from an old, soft woolen blanket.

Diapers: Four dozen diapers, two dozen 24-inch, two dozen 30-inch, are convenient. For the first few weeks, provided it is not hot weather, diapers 18 inches square, of old, soft, knitted wear, are very convenient. Several pieces of old sheeting torn into pieces 10 inches square may be put inside.

When diapers are removed, they should be put into a covered pail of cold water to which borax has been added. Later they should be washed clean with a pure soap, boiled, rinsed thoroughly, but not blued, and hung in the sun to dry. Soap and blueing are very irritating to a baby's skin. They should be folded, pressed with a hot iron, and put away. A soiled or wet diaper should *never be used a second time without being washed.* The urine contains substances which are very irritating to the skin of a baby.

Slips: For every-day wear there should be six plain white slips. These should be cut by the kimono-sleeve pattern and a tape run through a facing around the neck and sleeves.

If they are made 21 inches long from shoulder to hem, they will not need shortening. They should never be made longer than 27 inches. Two Sunday slips may be made with bishop sleeves and a little embroidery on the front. Set-in sleeves are more difficult to put on a little baby. For wear under the slips, baby needs also four flannel skirts, princess style. For hot weather these may be made of the very lightest weight flannel or part flannel and cotton.

Jackets: For cool mornings, baby needs three short jackets. These are made of white flannel over the kimono-sleeve pattern, or they may be knitted or crocheted with close stitches. There should be no loose stitches or scallops or other trimmings to catch on buttons or the baby's s fingers.

Out-of-door garments: The healthy baby is taken out of doors, so he must have a wrap and hood. This wrap is made like the sleeping bag except it is of white eiderdown or flannel. It may be sewed together or bound around with ribbon. At four months the upper corners may be opened so as to allow the baby to get its hands out freely. When baby begins to walk a very comfortable coat may be made from the bag. Open it and hem it at the bottom, shape the top loosely by a kimono-slip pattern.

For winter the hood may be made of the same material as the wrap, or it may be knitted or crocheted. For summer a silk or cotton knitted or crocheted hood of an open-lace pattern and lined with the very thinnest white silk is comfortable. Wash hoods may be made of soft white embroidered lawn and laundered without starch. The ties on the hood should be such as can be laundered easily. A little chin strap fastened at one side of the hood with a snap or hook and eye is very convenient and does away with the bow under the baby's chin.

Sleeping garments: Baby needs four "nighties" or sleeping bags of white outing flannel or knitted material. For winter wear the sleeves off the nightie may be made two inches longer, and the bottom eight inches longer. Draw tapes may be run through the sleeves, and tithe hem and baby's hands and feet thus protected from the cold.

Sleeping bags are made thirty-three inches long and twenty-seven inches wide, open down the front. The baby is laid in and the bag buttoned up. He can be changed without taking him out of the bag.

Woolen garments: All woolen or part-woolen garments must be washed very carefully. They should be washed by hand in tepid soapsuds (mild soap), rinsed in a little soapy water, and hung in the shade to dry. When dry, they should be pulled or patted into shape or smoothed with a warm iron before being put away. Always before putting garments on a baby they should be held to the cheek to be sure they are dry and warm.

Teething

When the baby comes into the world it is apparently toothless. Nevertheless, at this time the first teeth are practically completely formed, lying beneath the gums. In fact, under these first teeth there are already the beginnings of the permanent teeth. It needs no lengthy explanations to prove that these teeth cannot develop as they should if the body is not supplied a sufficient amount of the necessary building material. Hence, in the food for the child we should look especially to that part which builds bony structure, of which the tooth is a type. The two most important of these are phosphates and lime; and for the growing child there is no better source of these important elements than milk—mother's milk in infancy and clean cow's milk later. After infancy the diet of every child should include a glass of milk with each meal and in addition to this there should be other sources of mineral salts, such as fruits, green vegetables and pure water.

Teething a normal function: Teething in a healthy child is itself a normal function. It is only when associated with outside disturbances, especially with those due to indigestion or other abnormal conditions, that it may become a source of serious trouble, or when the teeth grow faster than the overlying tissues are absorbed to make room for them. There may then ensue sometimes very serious disturbances from the pressure of the tense and swollen gum on the coming crown underneath, which may, in some cases, be at once relieved by lancing the gum. If baby is sick, or has fever or loose bowels, do not attribute it to teething, but go to a doctor and find out what is the matter.

Order in which the teeth appear: Some time about the end of the sixth month, if the baby has been thriving normally, the first teeth, usually the lower front ones, that were lodged in baby's little jaws when it was born, will appear; and these will be followed at more or less regular intervals by the upper "incisors," then the "back teeth," and lastly, usually by the "cuspids," or, as they are popularly called, the "stomach" and the "eye" teeth.

The following gives approximately the time when these teeth usually break through the gums:

Two lower front teeth, at five to seven months.

Two upper front teeth, at six to eight months.

Two more lower front teeth, at seven to nine months.

Two more upper front teeth, at eight to ten months.

Four back (molar) teeth, one on each side of each jaw, at ten to fourteen months.

Four more molar teeth, back of the others, at about two years.

Four cuspids ("eye" and "stomach" teeth), at two to two and one-half years.

Every tooth, as it comes into place, is a milestone that marks another step in the child's development. It will not be until the cutting of all of its firsts full set of teeth has been completed that the mother may feel at liberty to give the child hard, solid food.

There are twenty of these first or milk teeth, ten in each jaw. As a help in remembering the baby teeth, recall that there are as many teeth in the upper jaw as there are fingers on two hands; and that a baby has as many teeth on the lower jaw as he has toes.

The time of cutting teeth varies so in different children that it is difficult to lay down rules for their appearance. However, a child one year of age has, as a rule, eight teeth; at sixteen months there should be twelve teeth, and at two and one-half years the child should have the full twenty. If the child has less than this number, there may be something lacking in the diet.

Proper food for sound teeth: Because of the effect of usage on the development of the teeth, it is clear that food should be presented in such form that it will require chewing. For this reason the diet should include a certain amount of coarse material for the purpose, especially, of exercising the teeth. Coarse whole-grained breads, fresh apples and similar articles included in the diet will do much to insure good teeth.

Toothbrush. The health of the second teeth depends much upon the care given the first set. As soon as they make their appearance, baby's teeth should be cleaned each day with a soft cloth or brush. When he is old enough, the child should be taught the daily use of the toothbrush.

Dental attention. The first teeth are necessary to hold the proper shape of the jaw until the second teeth are ready to break through. For that reason they should not be neglected. At the first sign of decaying teeth the child should be taken to a dentist.

The first set of teeth is replaced by the permanent teeth, beginning with the sixth year. The six-year molar may be recognized as the sixth tooth, counting from the midline of the jaw in front toward the back. Because this tooth comes through at the time the child is losing its temporary teeth it is often mistaken for one of them and is allowed to remain untreated and to decay. It is especially desirable that a child should be taken to a dentist at this time, because the six-year molar is one of the most important of all the teeth.

It sometimes happens that the first teeth are so firm that they do not fall out, but remain in the jaws and crowd back the second teeth, making them come in misshapen and irregular. Irregular teeth and resulting condition of the jaw may be remedied when a child is young.

Beautiful teeth are the right of every person.   Sound teethh are necessary to good health.

Keeping the Baby Well

To keep a baby well is much easier than to cure him when he becomes sick.

In a room crowded with strange people there always is likely to be someone who is suffering from a "catching" disease or who may have comes from a home where such a disease is present. For that reason a little baby should be kept away from crowds and from crowded places in order to protect him from exposure to disease.

Most healthy grown persons carry disease germs in their rmouths. They do an adult no harm. But in kissing a baby on the mouth these germs maty be transferred to the baby's tender mouth aind make him ill or even kill him. Kissing the baby on the mouth, even by his own mother, should not be permitted.

A *little cold* in a big person is likely to mean a *big cold* in a little baby. Anyone suffering from a cold, cough or sore throat should remain away from a young child. If the nursing mother catches a cold she should spray her nose and throat with an antiseptic solution and take every precaution against infecting her little one.

Whooping cough is another very dangerous disease for young children. Each year 10,000 or more young children died of this disease, the greater number of them being babies under three years of age - If the whooping cough does not kill, the long period of coughing, lasting sometimes for months, makes the child so weak and ill that he takes other diseases more readily.

Tuberculosis. All children are extremely susceptible to tuberculosis. To children under three years of age it is especially fatal. Few infants survive when suckled by tuberculous mothers. Breathing or coughing in the baby's face, kissing the baby, and the use of the same eating utensils are some of the commoner methods of infection. Children born guarded against infection, and if possible should be removed from such opportunity of contact.

Other dangerous diseases fro young children are measles, diphtheria and scarlet fever. Often they leave children suffering from sore eyes, running ears or other permanent injuries; and always the younger the child, the greater the chances he will die.

To keep a baby well, give him regular, systematic care, keep him away from crowds and away from sick people and every possible exposure to sickness or disease.

Symptoms of Sickness

The baby is sick if he has—

(1) No appetite.
(2) Vomiting.
(3) Diarrhea; or if the movements are slimy, frothy, bloody or contain particles of undigested food.
(4) Constipation; less than one good movement a day.
(5) Fever.
(6) Rash.
(7) Signs of a cold, sore throat, cough or discharges from the eyes and nose.
(8) Sweating of the head, especially if accompanied by restlessness and crying at night.
(9) Loss of weight or failure to gain properly.

What to Do for Any Sick Baby

(1) Give him an abundance of fresh air.
(2) Undress him and put him quietly to bed.
(3) Sponge with tepid water if he is feverish.
(4) Give little or no food, but plenty of pure, cool water.
(5) Send for the doctor. *The baby is sick enough to need medicine, he is sick enough to have a doctor give it.*

Sick room. If is possible to provide it, every home should contain one sunny bedroom with plain or washable walls and furniture, without carpels or draperies, that can be used as an isolation sick room in case of illness or emergency.

In *giving* the *following* list of home remedies and first-aid ttreatments it must be distinctly understood that the measures are to be undertaken only in an emergency pending the arrival of the doctor.

Whenever baby ill be sure to call promptly on the doctor for advice. Neglect of proper medical care is dangerous and responsible for the death of many babies.

Burns or Scalds. Other than small and light burns, send for a physician. The child may die from shock.

Emergency treatment. Remove clothing by cutting where necessary. Avoid dirty ointments or oils because of the danger of infection. Apply to burn as quickly as possible several layers of ssort cloth wet with solution of baking soda. Keep air away from burn.

Colds. Rest in bed as long as there is fever. Give less food and give only fruit juices and more water. Open the bowels freely with oil laxative. For complicated persistent or repeated colds, improve hygiene to build up the child's resistance, and apply to physician for treatment. Consult a surgeon for adenoids and diseased tonsils.

Constipation: The diet or habits are at fault. There may be a deficiency in the amount of fat in the diet, too much or too little sugar, or not enough fruit and green vegetables. A deficiency in the amount of water given is sometimes responsible. Do not give laxatives habitually; they make constipation worse. Send the child to stool at a regular time each morning. Use enema of one-half to one ounce of olive oil.

Convulsion: Without stopping to undress, place child in a tub bath, temperature 98 deg. F. (blood heat) for ten minutes. Always test water with your own bare elbow. Keep cold cloth around head and neck. If convulsions are caused by eating improper food, give prompt enema and laxative and warm-water emetic. Keep the child in bed until he recovers from shock. Consult a physician.

Cough: Avoid cough syrups; they are dangerous for children. Plain honey or stewed fig juice is soothing. Apply cold press to throat and chest. Ask the doctor to find the cause and follow his directions.

Croup: A child subject to repeated attacks of croup should be examined by a nose and throat specialist, and any treatment necessary to improve the health undertaken.

If breathing is difficult give warm salt or soda water emetic to induce vomiting.   Apply heat to the chest for ten minutes, followed by cold compress. If severe, throw a light blanket over child's head and the spout of kettle of boiling water, allowing child to inhale steam.

Croup which develops suddenly in a child previously well is not likely to be a serious matter. On the other hand, croup which develops slowly in a child previously ailing may be due to the formation of a diphtheritic membrane in the windpipe. No time should be lost in calling a doctor.

Crying: The very sick baby does not cry hard. There is a low moaning or wail, with sometimes a turning of the head from side to side. A whimpering, crying baby is hungry, or may be suffering from indigestion. A fretful crying baby is sleepy or uncomfortable. Lusty crying may be temper. Crying with tears in the eyes and clenching of the fists indicates pain. Irritability and lustful crying at night may be a symptom or scurvy. When that condition is present, handling is usually painful to the child. A mother should learn to recognize the nature of baby's cry.

Diarrhea: In babies diarrhea is due to incorrect feeding or to contaminated food. Stop all food for twelve hours. Begin again to feed with diluted milk no solid food for several days.

Give baby all he wants of cool boiled water. If you are far away from a doctor or can't get one immediately, give the baby a teaspoonful of fresh castor oil.   *Do not give him patent medicines or mixtures advised by neighbors.*

Dog or cat bite: Send for a doctor. Do not kill the animal but pen and observe it for symptoms of rabies. Extract poison from wound, applying warm water to make it bleed more freely. If dog is undoubtedly mad, the wound must be cauterized with strong nitric acid or hot iron. Telegraph to the State Board of Health at once for directions for securing treatment.

Drowning: Do not stop for anything, but at once suspend the child's head downward and pull tongue forward to allow water to run out of mouth. Lay the patient face down, the tongue out, and do artificial respiration for several hours. (See any standard text on first aid.) Put warm blankets about the child and rub arms and legs toward heart. Get a doctor as soon as possible.

Earache: Symptoms of earache in infants: Crying, turning the head from side to side, trying to put the hand on aching side. Earache very frequently accompanies or follows a severe cold or an attack of tonsillitis, and then is caused by an extension of the inflammation to the middle ear. This may result in deafness or mastoid abscess. Apply dry heat hot water bottle or dry salt heated and placed in a sack or old sock. Drop into the ear a few drops of five per cent phenol in glycerine. Never neglect earache. Have the child examined by a doctor, and if necessary by an ear specialist.

Eyes (sore or inflamed): Sore eyes are reportable by law. Call your doctor. While waiting for him to come, bathe the eyes hourly with a saturated solution of boric acid.

Eczema: Cleanse affected parts with olive oil, avoiding water, soap or other irritating substance. In eczema the diet is usually at fault. Keep the bowels open freely. Apply remedies and change the diet according to physician's directions.

Fainting: Place child with head lower than the rest of the body. Get fresh air. Dash cold water on face. Rub extremities toward heart. If fainting is frequent, consult a physician.

Fever: Fever is not a disease but a symptom. Undress and put the child to bed. Reduce diet and give plenty of drinking water and fruit juices. Open the bowels. Apply cool cloths to head and neck or give cool or tepid sponge baths. In high temperature, 103 deg. or over, or continued or frequent temperature, send for the doctor.

Foreign body in ear. Do not attempt to remove by poking. Lay the side of the head with the affected ear down and wait for the doctor. If a live insect has crawled into the ear, put into the ear a few drops of sweet oil or mineral oil.

Foreign body in eye: Tears may wash it out. Do not rub the eye. If visible, remove with corner of clean handkerchief. Wash eye with boric acid solution. Consult a physician or eye specialist.

Foreign body in nose: Do not attempt to remove by poking. Let the child blow the nose while holding the opposite nostril shut. If this fails, call the doctor.

Foreign body in throat: Do not get excited. Put your fingers in throat and remove the article. If you cannot reach it, hold child up by the ankles, head downward, and slap on the back. Then try reaching the obstruction again, if necessary. If the article has been swallowed, give the child a quantity of soft bread. Do not give laxative. Watch the stools for a few days. In most cases a foreign body will be passed without trouble.

Frostbite: Apply snow or ice to frostbitten parts. Keep child away from heat. Removal to warm room should be made with great care. For severe frostbite or freezing, call a physician.

Headache: Find out and treat cause. Headache may be due to constipation, indigestion, eye strain, excitement, fatigue or over-eating. Apply cold cloths to forehead and back of neck. Avoid headache remedies. They are exceedingly dangerous for children.

Holding the breath: Occurs after great excitement, crying or exposure to cold air. Dash cold water in face. If frequent, consult physician.

Night terrors: Probably caused by indigestion and constipation. Give the child a careful diet, light evening meal, healthy outdoor life, avoiding excitement. If continued or frequent, consult physician. Examine for enlarged tonsils, adenoids, decayed teeth, genital adhesions or tuberculosis.

Poisons swallowed: Better prevented than cured. Never put any poison where a child may possibly get into it. Learn the antidote for the commoner forms of poisoning, or keep a table of poisons and remedies. Always send for a doctor promptly, advising him of the poison taken so he may come prepared.

Insect stings: Remove the sting and apply spirits of camphor ammonia or wet baking soda.

Snake bite: The wound must be made to bleed freely, and poison must be sucked out. If a poisonous snake, tie a cord above wound to stop progress of the blood, and keep poison out of general circulation. Send for a doctor.

Sunburn: Prevent as much as possible by shade and by protecting the skin with cold cream before taking the child into the sun or wind. Avoid use of water on a sunburn. Apply sweet cream, almond lotion or cold cream.

Sore throat: Indicated in an infant by difficulty and pain in swallowing. Safest to call a physician. An older child may gargle the throat or have it sprayed with a mild antiseptic solution, such as one-fourth teaspoonful of baking soda and table salt to one cup of warm water. Sterilize drinking cup and tableware used by child with sore throat to prevent the spreading of the infection.

Sun prostration: Characterized by prostration, flushed face (sometimes pale and clammy) and vomiting. Requires only rest in cool room and tepid sponging.

Toothache: Clean cavity of all debris; pack decayed tooth with a bit of absorbent cotton with oil of cloves or five percent phenol in glycerine. Consult dentist always.

Vomiting (active): May be due to acute indigestion, infectious diarrheal disease or general infectious disease, scarlet fever or other acute eruptive disease. Stop giving food and water.

Habitual vomiting: Habitual vomiting may be caused by too rapid feeding, feeding in a reclining position or not holding the baby and bottle properly; laying the baby down too soon; rough handling of the baby too soon after feeding; wrong kind of food, particularly too much fat, sugar, or curd in raw milk; too large a total quantity at a feeding; too short intervals between feedings. Regulate faults of feeding. If vomiting is persistent, consult a physician.

Special Direction For Mothers Who Wish To Rear Their Children On Raw Food Diet

Every day after the fourth day give thirty minutes before second and fifth feedings one-half teaspoon of orange juice diluted with two ounces of water. This can be given to a breastfed baby with a teaspoon, a little at a time, or to a bottle-fed baby in a bottle same as milk. Increase to one teaspoonful orange juice until the baby is six weeks old.

FROM SIX WEEKS TO SIX MONTHS give: one teaspoon of orange juice with one teaspoon of spinach juice, alternated with lettuce juice and diluted with two ounces of water. Give this twice a day before second and last feeding.

After six weeks the mother may also at one feeding, on alternate days, add to the baby's milk, cereal water made from ground cereal soaked overnight and strained. Substitute two ounces of this for the milk.

AFTER THE SIXTH MONTH the baby can be given salads three times a day. At the meal when salad is given the milk should be reduced three ounces, but at other milk feedings should be given full quantity.

Salads should consist of one under-ground and one over-ground vegetable in this proportion. To two table-spoons of finely-chopped lettuce or spinach, add one teaspoon of grated carrot, beet or other underground vegetable. To this add one teaspoon of orange juice and one or two teaspoons of water.

Continue this diet with variety, increasing amount as the baby grows, until the baby's teeth have developed. While the teeth are coming in and the baby is fretful from irritated gums, don't give it teething rings and other devices to bite on. A silver spoon can be given the baby to play with, on which it will bite from time to time. The best thing to do is to take a young carrot, boring a hole through the upper part and put a string through this, hanging it around the baby's neck and allowing it to bite on that. Or give a piece of tender celery to bite on. In addition to allaying the irritation of the gums, the child receives the benefit of the live minerals which will aid in building the teeth and nerves ALWAYS USE SAME PROPORTION for salad, increasing salad only as the child grows and requires more food.

Something for mothers to remember. At the age of four months a child was brought to Dr. E. J. Dirinkall (who has been having uniform success in rearing and treating children with raw food) suffering from a severe cold, in the first stages of pneumonia and in a critical condition. It was immediately taken off all food and given one teaspoon each of orange and spinach juice with two ounces of water in place of food at each feeding. On this diet, after four days all symptoms of the disease, including the cold, disappeared, and the child gained rapidly in health and strength. This child had previously been fed on condensed milk exclusively.

A remedy for disease is simple when you resort to natural methods.

Grated sweet potato can be given for diarrhea.

Use small quantities of onion in salads occasionally. If the mother has no device for extracting juice it can be extracted from leafy vegetables by chopping fine and putting into a cheesecloth and squeezing through.

After the child has developed its teeth it should be given the vegetable salads, sliced or chopped, so as to give it an opportunity to use its teeth, and should be carefully watched by the mother to see that it learns to masticate properly, chewing the food to a creamy mass before swallowing.

From this time soon the child can be given its cereal at breakfast, ground in dry form and sprinkled over raisins or any fruit, and can partake of its meals the same as adults who are living on a raw food diet, except that the child's food should be regulated as to quantity.

One to two teaspoonfuls of nuts should be flaked and sprinkled over the salad once a day.

If the child is allowed to eat bread, never combine the bread with any acid fruit at the same meal.

At eight months begin to teach the child to drink from a cup.

Children should drink plenty of water all through the day. At meals, if water or milk is given, teach them to drink a small amount at one time only after it has swallowed its thoroughly masticated food.

Mothers should be careful not to create a desire for unnatural sweets which later develop a craving for candy other than that made from pure material, which we already know from other articles in this book has a detrimental effect on the child's health. Teach it instead to want fruits in their natural state, and for sweets let it have dates, figs, etc. Develop a love for all healthful play and exercise and all things pertaining to nature.

A child fifteen months old and at present living on the alternating diet given below was taken for treatment while in a serious condition, by Dr. E. J. Drinkall of Chicago when five days old. It was highly irritable, unable to retain its food, its energy and vitality so low that there was little hope of saving its life.

The child was taken off all forms of food and placed upon juices as described, and as its health increased milk was added. At six months it was placed upon this diet, adhering to it daily with its variations up to the present time, and is now a robust, healthy child, full of life and energy and has a wonderful disposition. It has been free from children's diseases, is never irritable, sleeps soundly and is always happy. This is one of the many examples showing what raw food will do for your baby.

> 6 A. M. —Flaked natural peanuts—two teaspoons. Chopped lettuce (fine)—half cup. Grated beet—one teaspoon. Orange juice—one teaspoon. Water—two teaspoons. Fresh whole milk—six ounces.
>
> 9 A. M. —Fresh whole milk—nine ounces.
>
> 12 P.M. —Same vegetable combination without the nuts. Fresh whole milk—six ounces.
>
> 3 P. M. — Fresh whole milk—nine ounces.
>
> 6 P. M. — Same vegetable combination as at breakfast without nuts. Fresh whole milk—six ounces.

Cabbage is used in place of lettuce.

Celery, cabbage is used in place of lettuce.

A teaspoon of finely-chopped spinach is used several times a week.

Carrots, turnips, parsnips and sweet potato are alternated with the beet.

In the summer season tomato can be used with one of the leafy above-ground vegetables. No orange juice to be used with tomato juice or tomato.

The quantity at all times will be guided and governed by the capacity of the child to be fed.

To 2 ounces macerated banana add 1 teaspoon of flaked nuts (Apple may be substituted for banana)

This makes a wholesome and nutritious dish for the baby after it begins eating solid food.

A Nourishing Nut Milk for the Baby

Nut milk is splendid for building the body of baby, child and adult. But caution should be exercised in feeding it to the undernourished baby, as it is powerful in proteins. It is best to use it after the undernourished child begins to build and then not more frequently than every other day.

Take one, two or three tablespoonfuls flaxseed to a cup of filtered rain water. Let soak one hour and stir every ten minutes. Then add spinach, orange or lettuce juice in equal amounts to the liquid flaxseed. Add one ounce of flaked Pignolias or Peanuts mixed together and strain through a small strainer.   Sweeten to taste with honey.

Estes and Drews.

It will do no harm to leave flaxseed in the milk. The amount of flaxseed used is optional.

Nut Emulsion

Mix and rub into a butter one ounce of Pignolias or Peanuts flaked very fine and one-half ounce of waiter. Mix into this butter, little by little, six ounces water; beat it briskly with a rotary eggbeater and pour it through a large tea strainer. Stir it when it clogs the strainer. Add to this emulsion, at your option, one-half ounce honey (teaspoonful) and serve in a glass with a teaspoon or rye straw.

Drews.

Imitation Buttermilk

Put into a cup cone-half ounce flaxseed and add six ounces waiter. Beat it briskly with a rotary eggbeater every ten minutes during one hour. Meanwhile mix and rub together three-fourths ounce lemon juice (three tea-spoonfuls) and ounce pignolias or peanuts flaked very fine or twice. Let this stand fifteen minutes or so; then add to it the above flaxseed fluid and beat it very briskly with the rotary beater. Now pour it through a large tea strainer, stir to prevent clogging, and serve in a glass with a teaspoon or rye straw. This is cooling in summer and refreshing in winter.

Drews.

Near Milk

Near milk is prepared like near buttermilk, with the exception that in place of the rhubarb juice only pure water or orange juice is used. This milk is wholesome, delicious, appetizing, cooling and refreshing. All the infectious diseases, such as consumption, lumpjaw and several fevers which may be transmitted to man in cow's milk, are barred out of near milk.

Drews.

Near Buttermilk

Soak in a cup three-fourths full of water one ounce flaxseed and beat it about every ten minutes during the course of one hour with a rotary eggbeater. Before beating the last time fill the cup nearly full with water and then let the seed settle. Meanwhile mix and rub into a cream one ounce pignolias or peanuts flaked exceedingly fine and one-half ounce of rhubarb juice. Put this cream into a cup and add three and one-half ounces flaxseed fluid and beat it again briskly. Now pour it through a large tea strainer, stirring the while to keep it from clogging. Serve in a glass with a teaspoon or rye straw. At your option you may add a half ounce honey (teaspoonful).

Drews.

"Lemonized" Milk

Into a cup containing six ounces sweet milk pour three-fourths ounce lemon juice (or half a lemon) and beat it briskly with a rotary egg-beater for two minutes to prevent it from curdling in lumps. This milk is acid sterilized. It is more wholesome for weaned children and adult convalescents than warm or sweet milk. Milk is not advised in the natural diet, but if it must be used let it be "lemonized" milk.

Drews.

IRIOLOGY

A comparatively new science is the study of disease as revealed by the human eye. It has been proved that every disease known to the human family manifests itself in the eyes in colors and characteristic markings. This science is called Iriology and Iridiagnosis.

Before long this study will have been so perfected that the physician will be capable of diagnosing diseases long before any symptoms have become apparent.

Such diseases as rheumatism, neuritis, cancer, anemia, spinal disorders, kidney trouble, diseases of the jaws and the teeth, ulcers, liver disturbances and gastro-intestinal infections may be diagnosed by the eye.

It would seem, then, most important that everyone familiarize himself to as great an extent as possible with the facts concerning Iriology and Iridiagnosis.

Because the science is of recent origin and demands detailed observation and study, its followers are limited at the present time. Iriology possesses great possibilities as an aid to medical science, and the remarkable progress achieved by those who have followed it as a profession has already gained wide recognition.

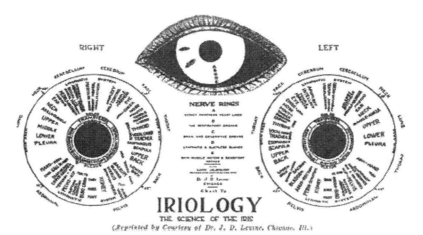

IRIOLOGY
THE SCIENCE OF THE IRIS
(Reprinted by Courtesy of Dr. J. D. Levine, Chicago, Ill.)

Raw Food and Health

The founder of Iriology was Dr. Ignatz Peczely of Budapest Hungary. As a small boy eleven years of age while playing in his father's garden he captured an owl. In the struggle one of the owl's legs was broken, and the boy subsequently noted a white cloud in the lower part of the iris on the side corresponding to the iris on the side corresponding to the broken leg. After the leg healed the boy again examined the owl's iris and noticed that a black speck, circumscribed by white lines, had replaced the former cloudlike sign.

When Peczely reached manhood he took up the study of medicine, and it was during his practice years later that he was called upon to treat a man's fractured leg. He recalled the incident of the owl and forthwith examined his patient's eye. The experience with the owl was repeated, for he found a curious mark in the patient's eye which greatly resembled that which he had observed in the bird's.

Persistent observation and study enabled Peczely to discover various areas in the eye which definitely corresponded to the organs of the body, and thus the foundation for Iriology and Iridiagnosis was established.

Peczely first and only was published in 1880 in Budapest, Hungary. Numerous followers appeared m Europe. Dr Henry Lane, Dr. Henry Lindlahr, Dr. J D. Levine, Dr. J. Dequer and Dr. J. H. Kritzer are among those who have successfully practiced Iriology in the United States.

Dr. Lane of Chicago (now departed), under whom Dr. J, D. Levine studied, did valiant work for the science of Iriology, but for some reason, whether from personal modesty or lack of appreciation by those in the profession, his services have failed to receive the mention which they so fully deserve, and his important contributions to science have been somewhat obscured.

The normal eye is smooth and silky-looking in texture, with no lines, spots or fibers marring the surface.

Aristotle (400 B. C.) was probably the first to discover that the color of the iris in the new-born was blue. This has been verified by leading scientists and physicians throughout the world in the evolution of the human race.

The light blue eye or the light brown eye indicates a healthy condition. The lighter the eye, the cleaner the body, the light, clear eye indicates that the ductless glands are draining off the poisons of the body.

Only about ten percent of the human race is born with a natural brown eye, and this is a racial characteristic, a condition of toxic poison which is transmitted from one generation to the next. These natural brown eyes are found in extremely dark-skinned types, particularly Armenians, Turks, etc.

Toxic poisons and drugs are responsible for the changes in color and the markings of the eye.

The classification of the eye are:
1. Clear blue, whitish blue, grayish blue and inky blue.
2. Clear brown, amber brown or muddy brown, dark brown and roasted coffee brown.
3. Intermediate. This is a hybrid shade of an indistinct color, bluish brown, or brownish blue of light and dark shades of a greenish cast, according to the dominant shade of blue making for the lighter or the dominant brown making for the darker shade.
4. Mixed colors. To this class are assigned all irides which were originally blue or brown, but have changed in parts due to the deposit in the system of various crude drugs, making for the yellow or "cat-eye," orange and steel gray shades and many so-called brown or hazel irides.
5. The pink, or albino iris, is found in people who are unusually fair, almost white; hence the desig-

nation "albino"—alba, Latin for white—which is
due to a lack of pigmentation in the lining of the
choroid at the back of the eye so that light passing
through the iris and pupil is tinged red from the
blood vessels at the back, thus their eyes may
seem to "blush simultaneously with their face."

All men who are administering drugs of a poisonous
character should thoroughly understand the systemic
changes taking place within the body by the use of those
drugs. It seems from the research that has been done along
these lines that there is not any drug that has been administered but will show its effect in the iris of the eye, and
iridiagnosis proves conclusively that when a patient recovers from the illness resulting from vaccines and drugs
which have been administered he is only relieved of the
symptoms and not of the potential cause. The eye proves
conclusively that the crude, poisonous drugs are not eliminated from the system. For this reason it is well that
dentists familiarize themselves with this form of diagnosis,
especially where they are using, in some cases, excessive
amounts of arsenic and iodine in tooth and gum treatments
and different forms of drugs and strong solutions upon the
mouth and tissues.

The whitish blue or whitish gray iris denotes acidosis,
which is due to an excessive accumulation of various acids,
particularly uric acid, in the blood and tissues.

The darkening of the whitish blue or the whitish gray
iris denotes a subacute form of acidosis.

In the brown iris, acidosis produces the amber color of a
cloudy appearance.

These findings are based upon the fact that in every
case the patient has subsisted upon acid-producing foods,
such as meat, eggs, white bread, white sugar, tea and
coffee.

Observation also disclosed that the iris cleared up after the patient had suffered an acute attack of arthritis or some other disease which cleared the system of the acids and the iris of the milky covering. Also, that the iris cleared following a change in diet from the cooked, acid-producing foods and restriction to a diet of fresh fruits and green, leafy vegetables, rich in organic mineral salts, thus neutralizing and eliminating the acids from the system.

It must be remembered that every organ has its exact corresponding area in the iris. These become visible only through abnormal changes—pathological or functional disturbances—taking place in such organs.

"Scurf rim" is a term used to indicate abnormal functions and structure of the skin, as revealed in the iris. It is a Greek word, "scorbutus," meaning scurvy, and as it surrounds the iris it is called a rim. It shows a partial or complete dark covering of the periphery of the iris and is formed in pyorrhea cases, measles, chicken pox and numerous other conditions where lowered circulation and depleted health have impaired the normal functions of the skin.

Only those ingredients which are neither assimilated nor eliminated by the body are manifested in the iris.

Sodium, or table salt, and other inorganic salts, form a whitish or silver gray ring of metallic luster in the eye. This may indicate:

1. That the patient is subject to rheumatism and has been treated with sodium salicylate.
2. Acidity of the stomach. Remedy taken, sodium bicarbonate.
3. Excess consumption of baking soda in bread, cakes, biscuit, etc.
4. Excessive use of table salt.
5. Saline cathartics.

Arsenic shows white flakes in the eye.

Dr. Kritzer states observation has led him to believe that arsenic is more often found in the blue iris than brown—indicating that the blue is more susceptible to that drug.

Arsenic is used as a heart and brain stimulant, for gastric disorders, bronchial and respiratory diseases, malaria, skin eruptions, cancer and in syphilis treatment, in treatment of the teeth, etc.

Phosphorus shows white flakes similar to arsenic. Phosphorus deposits anywhere in the iris. It afflicts the abdomen, back, jaws and diaphragm; also the heart. Phosphorus may be absorbed through inhalation and phosphorus poison, which manifests itself in. the form of *necrosis of the jaw,* is common to workers in match factories. Phosphorus poison produces fatty degeneration. Phosphorus is given as an alternative in softening of the bones (osteo malacia), rickets and in neurosis as general nerve tonic. It is also given for sexual impotence. Its temporary stimulating action is followed by permanent ill effects.

Creosote shows sparkling white spots in the eye around the pupil. Creosote is used in respiratory disorders, tuberculosis, mouth washes, root canal purifiers, etc. It is obtained by the distillation of wood-tar.

Quinine is used in manufacture of aspirin, given as tonic, also used in rheumatism, tonsillitis, neuralgia, typhoid, etc. Causes roaring in the ears, deafness, blindness and headaches. Yellowish green, greenish yellow color in the eye, commonly called "cat eye."

Sulphur shows a dark brown, cloud-like discoloration. It is used in laxatives, tonics, skin diseases, sulphur vapor baths; the inhalation of sulphur in these vapor baths greatly impairs the health.   Another source of sulphur poison is found in sulphur-cured fruits, and grains from which flour is made.

Lead is used as a local sedative and astringent, internally as astringent and hemostatic. Lead preparations are used in skin diseases, ear troubles, diarrhea and vaginal douches. Chronic poison develops through the absorption of lead in face powders, tooth pastes, cosmetics. Lead poison shows characteristic softening of gums and a blue pencil line along margin of teeth.

Iodine shows red spots surrounded by white borders. It is found in any area of the iris. It deposits in any region of low vitality, according to Iridiagnosis. It is used as an antiseptic, germicide and counter-irritant for various inflammatory conditions, particularly of the gums and teeth, joints, pleura, lymph glands, goiters and in syphilis treatment.

Salivation frequently results from iodine poisoning, due either to the irritating effect it has upon the salivary glands during active process of elimination or to the effect of the iodides upon systemic mercurial deposits resulting from medication. Mercury is kept in solution by the action of iodine.

Opium and Morphine show minute black lines in the eye around the pupil. They form a perfect wheel-like circle.

Ergot shows a reddish circle in the eye lighter than iodine. Ergot is used to bring on labor, stop hemorrhages and contract tissues and blood vessels. It weakens the muscles of the heart, blood vessels and muscle fibers of the stomach.

Coal Tar Products are recognized by the presence of a dark, dirty gray veil covering almost one half of the upper part of the iris.

Analgesics, anodyne (pain relievers), as well as various antipyretics, are classed among tar products. The numerous derivatives are acetanilid, aspirin, phenacetin, antipyrin, an-tikamnia, etc., all of which are found among the patent medicines given for headaches, toothaches, fevers and other ailments of nervous origin. Coal tar products may also be absorbed through the use of oil of wintergreen, cinnamon oil, lysol, salicylic acid, naphthol and benzol alcohol; also through extracts which are synthetically produced from crude oil and used in ice cream sodas, orangeades, pink lemonades and "doctored" cherries. The coloring matter of cheap candies and most of the preserved canned goods are prepared with coal tar products.

Saccharin, which is used as a substitute for sugar, is a coal tar product which in time has a most serious effect upon the brain and nervous system. Most cheap candies contain saccharin and coal tar dyes. These dyes, synthetic flavorings and saccharin form an important constituent in the manufacture of soft drinks. Some perfumes are of coal tar origin. Tomato catsup is preserved with anilin dye, which is a coal tar product.

Mercury shows in the eye in a whitish or silver-gray circular line of marked metallic luster. Where used in connection with potassium iodide, mercury may show like a sodium ring. It shows blue in the brown iris. The potassium iodide keeps the metallic salts soluble in the bloodstream. The presence of mercury in the system may not be detected for from five to fifteen years after its use. The circulation of this metallic salt in the arterial system gradually causes it to deposit itself in the walls of the blood vessels, resulting in hardening of the arteries, aneurism of the aorta or other valvular disease.

Mercury is used as a disinfectant, antiseptic and cautery. Its local use is as an astringent and irritant and for irrigation of the bodily cavities. It is also a base for silver fillings for the teeth, ointments, powders, rouges and is administered internally in the form of calomel.

For the benefit of the dentists who use a great many alloy fillings, it has been found that the alloy, coming in contact with the salt contained in the food, forms bichloride of mercury. The symptoms in such cases often manifest themselves in catarrhal irritation of the respiratory tract Sore and ulcerated gums, loose teeth (pyorrhea), necrosis of the jaws, inflammation of the salivary glands, anemia loss of flesh and strength and aching of the bones and joints are only a few of the results of mercurial poisoning.

The nervous system and brain are particularly susceptible to metal poisoning. Excitability and sclerosis in the brain are, according to authorities, manifestations of metallic poisoning. The iris substantiates this statement, especially with regard to mercury, as it has an affinity for the brain and spinal cord.

Dr. Kritzer cites the case of a young mother of two children, who developed extreme mental afflictions due to mercurial poisoning. She had been kept under mercurial treatment for five years on the mere suspicion of syphilis. The heavy ring in the iris told the story. Later the corroboration was furnished by the eruption of boils and a mercurial rash which developed under rational treatment.

Cessation of violent symptoms and a decrease of the mercurial sign was noted following proper treatment.

Vaccines show black or muddy brown spots surrounded by white borders. They are superficially deposited on the surface of the iris.

Dr. J. D. Levine states that his experience and research in Iriology has been of such an extensive character that he is able to judge the vitality of any person and whether that individual is still capable of fighting his condition or whether the physical conflict will exhaust him. He claims he has discovered the solar plexus region known as the abdominal brain, one of the most important nerve centers in the body. He has perfected a method whereby that region may be built up to function better. He also discovered the mental and memory centers of the brain as well as adhesions in the body, as shown in the iris.

Another discovery has been to tell the condition of the spinal column, whether it is rotated and which side to treat, regardless of the patient's symptoms.

Numerous demonstrations of Dr. Levine's ability to diagnose according to the conditions of the eye were confirmed by several of my own patients whom I sent to him. X-rays and case histories proved Levine's statements as to spinal, glandular and other disturbances.

Examination of one of many school children revealed an injury to the child's brain The mother was instructed to be prepared for convulsions. The mother told the doctor that the child has been subject to these convulsions, but as he appeared strong and healthy the parents thought he was feigning them to evade attending school.

Kidney stones, bladder diseases, uterine congestion, injuries to the face resulting in frontal sinus trouble, fallen stomach, the causes of colds, can all be diagnosed from the iris.

Dr. Levine states that seventy per cent of his cases suffering from colds require treatment of the stomach, intestines, liver or kidneys instead of the throat. The eye quickly tells what produced the cold.

One of the remarkable factors in this science of Iridiagnosis is the ability to tell the conditions of the teeth. Many a child has its teeth treated when the nose and throat should be looked after instead. Other cases of de-calsification and of caries (so the eye shows) are due to systemic poisons and glandular inactivity. The glands being tired out, do not detoxify or destroy the poisons in the body. Demineralization takes place, and the teeth crumble away, and all the dental work in the world will not save them for any protracted period.

Proper physical attention, elimination of the bodily poisons and foods, the vital foods, are more important, effective and permanent in correcting diseases than the drugs which cure or repress the symptom but leave the cause untouched.

Decay of the teeth shows in the iris in white or black lines, the white indicating acute inflammation or irritation, the black signifying a chronic state of inflammation or irritation.

When a real black spot appears in the iris, it means a lesion and indicates that some nerve center, organ or muscle is chronically affected.

A spot which is not black but deeper than the shade of the eye means the beginning of an irritated condition; it is a slight congested condition which is the pathological beginning of more serious developments to follow.

Conditions of the throat are usually due, not to congestion or lesions, but to some constitutional disorder, among which may be poor metabolism, taking place in people who eat improper foods and fail to assimilate properly, glandular disturbances, eye disorders, injuries to the neck and spine incurred through accidents or wrestling (frequently boys wrestling will twist and injure the neck and spine, weaken the nerves and cause congestion and nervous disorders), etc.

The poisons generated in the system as a result of these conditions send a backwash to the throat which weakens the nerves. This weakened condition affects the anterior muscles of the cervical region or in time produces a nerve contraction which has an irritating effect on the trifacial nerves. Chronic conditions of this nature culminate in a vicious cycle which has a definite effect on the teeth, and the teeth in turn affect the body.

There are practically no instances where the patients, according to the iris, have apparently good health and extensive tooth troubles. The tooth conditions are always apparent in the iris.

Few people are so healthy that the eye is perfect. Levine states that in the course of his experience he has found only two with clear, healthy eyes.

The blue eye does not necessarily mean power and strength. It more probably indicates freedom from toxic poisons, but an individual may have blue eyes with no lesions and still be afflicted with a very low vitality which is due to an inherited condition or to an injury which he has suffered to the solar plexus region or the sympathetic nervous system.

The person with clear blue or light brown eyes is less likely to succumb to the effects of an epidemic.

With the exceptions which have been mentioned, all people are born with blue eyes, even colored babies have a grayish-blue iris.

Most mountaineers and sailors have blue eyes. Their rugged outdoor life and the constant exposure tend to keep the system free from accumulated poisons which change the color of the iris.

Even kittens have blue eyes when first born.

Brown eyes only predominate in the crowded, congested cities, where fresh air, exercise and all factors conducive to health seem to be at a premium.

The foregoing are just the merest facts regarding the effects of the health upon the color of the eyes, but they may serve as an incentive for experiment by those who are interested in bettering their physical condition.

Although the eye is a small organ and only the colored area is used for diagnostic purposes, it is capable of revealing so many of the bodily conditions that we have not even touched upon the great possibilities of Iriology which the future will unfold. The science of Iriology is in its infancy. There is not anything miraculous about this new science. Does not the astronomer tell you the size of a star, how old it is and how fast it travels even if it be a million miles away and invisible to the naked eye?

HEALTH VS. VOICE

The technical training of a voice is exploited as an accomplishment. Singing is listed with the arts. It is a social enhancement, a professional asset but not generally regarded as an *adjunct* to *health.* This last is a feature of voice training which eludes notice, because the *effect* is what compels attention rather than the *cause.*

Everyone knows that singers as a class are very solicitous for their state of health and are constantly guarding against possible ills lest the voice be impaired in the slightest degree. Health is essential to a perfect voice, and likewise voice-training is conducive to better health. The successful singer has an open throat, clear air passages in the head, well developed and thoroughly oxygenated lungs and powerful muscles in the abdomen and diaphragm. These are all fundamentals for a voice, and if any one of these primary requisites is lacking, the voice will also lack either in power, resonance, control or feeling, and for the experienced ear it is not difficult to determine very quickly just which of these factors is missing.

Aside from these essentials, which are all valuable in building health as well as a voice, there is the reaction of almost the entire body.

Vocal exercises are given to the beginner to loosen the taut muscles of the face and the lips, to lend flexibility to the jaws, pliancy to the tongue. In conjunction with these are given exercises to relax the tension of the throat and increase the breathing capacity. Great stress is laid upon the posture of the body while singing. Chest and shoulders should be held up, the weight thrown on the balls of the feet instead of on the heels, the arms relaxed instead of rigidly held at the sides or behind the back. All these facts are emphatically important to the singer, not only as regards his appearance, but the actual production of tone.

When these salient points are regarded in connection with voice training, it will be easily understood how the entire body is subjected to the closest consideration and rigorous development, insofar as this development is related to production of a voice.

With few exceptions, the attention to the body is restricted to those organs which are directly affiliated with the voice, namely, the head, throat, chest, lungs, diaphragm and abdomen. Closest detailed study is given the respiratory organs. The attention to the other parts of the body is of a more or less superficial character.

Effects of health on the voice: The voice, whether it be speaker's or singer's—the lecturer's, orator's, actress' or grand opera star's —is based upon the state of health of that individual. No voice can be built without health, and no matter how beautiful and powerful the voice, it will not be long sustained if its possessor suffers a gradual physical depletion or an abrupt collapse.

Voice is an outward expression of an inward power; physical power, beauty of interpretation and comprehension of soul. A man may sing like an angel and act like a demon, but the fact that the beautiful, throbbing tones of his voice will sway an audience and move it to tears shows that that man has the quality of emotional feeding and the depth of soul which enables him to penetrate to the spark of Divine intelligence which stirs within us all.

If, then, this voice expression, with its resonance and vibration, is dependent upon the power and energy of its owner, which is an undeniable fact and is based on the simplest logic, how is this power to be built? The answer is obvious. We do not build skyscrapers on wobbly foundations; we do not construct dreadnaughts with beams and rivets of aluminum. Emphatically NO! We build foundations of rock, sink them hundreds of feet into the ground that they may be relied upon to support the monuments to commerce which rise like obelisks against the skies of our large cities. We use only the strongest iron, the most resistive metal known for practical use in constructing the men-of-war which breast the raging seas and defy our foes.

Hence, to build or sustain a voice, we must have a foundation of Health—the cornerstone of all power and achievement—Health in its truest, fullest sense, which means that the entire body with all its essential parts and co-relating organs, as nearly approaches 100% of perfection as it is possible for us to keep it. Most people exist; only a few really live. They content themselves with a haphazard mode of life, envy the occasional radiantly-healthy person they chance to meet and, so long as they are fortunate enough to keep out of the hospital, congratulate themselves on their general good luck. The sudden demise of an apparently healthy friend jars their serenity for a time, causes them some apprehension as to their own physical condition, but these fears subside as the days pass and are soon forgotten.

What real health is: Health doesn't mean that you are active and energetic two days in succession and dull and lethargic for four days afterward. Health doesn't mean a hearty appetite and subsequent indigestion and constipation. Health does not mean periodic fits of uncontrollable nervousness, alternate moods of hilarity and melancholia. In short, health is not a state in which some of the organs function all the time and all of the organs function some of the time. *Health,* real 100% health, is that state of body wherein *all* of the *organs* function *properly* all of the *time.*

"But," you may object, "that is perfection! We are human. We are subject to constant and relentless decomposition. We are not supposed to live forever."

All right! Did anybody, from Jesus Christ down to the keenest brain of the present day, ever tell you just how long you were supposed to live? I think not. The only basis you have to go on has been the precedent established by those who were too ignorant or too lazy to care for themselves and consequently passed out when they should have been just getting a good start in life. Isn't it a fact that the people whose lives are recorded in the Bible lived more than 50 or 60 years? Did anyone express any surprise and give a great celebration when a prophet or seer reached his hundredth birthday? We have no chronicles to that effect. Three-score and ten was the minimum—the rule, not the exception.

If you think God created you for the purpose of having you allow your body to pass into a state of decay before you are called upon to discard that body and pass into a higher state of vibration, you are sadly misinformed. God created man with a clean body, not one filled with impurities, and because at the beginning of the world man was endowed with the will to choose good or evil, he seems to utilize this power of selection for the speedy destruction of himself.

A clean, pure bloodstream is the only foundation for health. Without it, no real, lasting health can be built, regardless of all care, exercise and attention to the most minute detail. The bloodstream circulates through and nourishes every atom of the body, and if that bloodstream is clogged with impurities, laden with poisons, how in the name of all that is sane and sound, can it build a body to health? It is an utter impossibility, and the futility of it is being demonstrated every day by physicians who treat and treat and re-treat *symptoms* of diseases instead of the *causes* of the disease which have their source in the bloodstream.

"But," you may ask, "what is responsible for a diseased bloodstream?" Man and animals are born with a clean and sterile intestinal tract, minus the bacteria and the many micro-organisms found after they have matured. Manifestly these poisons and bacteria are generated by foreign matter taken into the body in the shape of food.

Cooked, demineralized foods are the certain agents of decomposition and putrefaction. They have no life in them, and the process of degeneration begins almost at once. If you set a dish of cooked food aside with a dish of the same food uncooked, you will find that *disintegration* of the cooked food is *immediately* begun, whereas the *raw food* endures for some time before actual decay is observed. Moreover, the odor of the decomposed cooked food will be extremely offensive and far more penetrating than the odor of the same food which has been allowed to decay without having first been cooked.

The fact that decomposition of the cooked food begins at once when it is set aside shows that the resistive forces of that food have been cooked out and it is open to the assaults of the bacteria, which cause fermentation and putrefaction. Since these cooked foods decay and become putrid in a short time when they are allowed to stand in a refrigerator or pantry, is it not logical that they putrefy and become foul with twice the rapidity when they are retained in the intestines along with the other accumulations? Certainly. There is no evading the issue.

It may occur to the reader that I am digressing from my subject, but I am not. I have that subject before me mentally, and I am purposely explaining (and repeating the explanation given in previous pages) the action of cooked food upon the body to show the importance of food to health; and since we have already proved that health must be the foundation of the voice, then we have the analogy of food to voice.

Poisons of food conveyed to blood. The poisons of the intestines generated by the cooked foods are absorbed into the bloodstream and ply their ruinous course through the entire body, feeding the myriads of nerves and tissues on poisonous blood, which is constantly increasing its noxious quality by the absorption of the foods which are eaten daily. With the persistent and long-continued use of cooked food, the blood is unable to purify itself and consequently carries to the cells a poisonous nourishment which has such a small percentage of the essentials of nourishment that the cells are forced to drag along as best they can and are finally obliged to draw on their reserve energy. This goes on all over the body until the reserve energy is consumed. Then commences the inevitable physical breakdown. Very gradually it comes on in some cases, abruptly in others, dependent upon the original strength of the constitution and the inherited resistance. Meanwhile, all during the time that the accumulated poisons have been laying waste to the body and lowering the vitality, diseases of the various organs have set in, frequently without the individual's knowledge. Thus, everything conspires to undermine the health, although the person, unconscious of his own culpability, aids and abets the degenerative process by continually feeding on cooked foods.   Hence, we have the cycle of life—the endless chain— until the untimely end.

And now that we have established the importance of health, and the necessity of a clean, pure bloodstream to maintain that health, let us consider the success of a voice as related to health. In referring to the voice, I mean the speaking *voice* as well as the singing voice, for health is essential to both, and it is important for everyone to *speak* correctly, even if he never develops the singing voice. Development and placement of a speaking voice is a great advantage to everyone, both as a personal asset and a conducive factor to health.

Great voices do not last: Having read this far, I am prepared to have my readers raise a question to the effect that the greatest voices of the world have been developed on a diet of cooked food. Very true. Ask yourself how long these same beautiful voices lasted. If the singers themselves did not die prematurely, as many have, their voices expired just when they were in the full bloom of maturity. Again, the objection comes, and the excuse, "overwork, over-taxation," etc., is offered. All right. If those singers had known the proper kind of food to live on, had understood what their bodies were capable of if nourished on life-giving foods, many of them would be alive today. They would not have succumbed to disease and death from strain and over-taxation. Caruso is in his grave today as a result of the foods he ate, and the world is deprived of a magnificent voice which should have charmed it for many years to come, instead of being stilled by death. Farrar retired a year ago at the height of her career because her health had failed and she was no longer able to reach the high tones which had so singularly distinguished her.

If the body is poisoned with cooked foods, the vitality is lowered and the nerves depleted. With these conditions the slightest over taxation induces serious trouble.

Anyone who has lost a voice may, if he is conversant with the elemental rules of Health, foods and regeneration of bodies, build himself to such strength and superb health that he can regain his voice by natural methods and build it to greater power and beauty than it formerly possessed.

Patti fasted a great deal of the time, thereby acknowl-edging her recognition of the destructive effects of excess food on the voice. In fact, all singers abstain from food for a number of hours before appearing before their audience. They also abstain from eating sweets, as the effect of the sugar on the delicate membranes of the throat produces a peculiar huskiness, or thickness, which mars the clarity of the voice.

Physically, singers are apt to be large and well formed, but this seems due chiefly to an inherited constitution rather than a result of physical culture, and the fact that enormous voices are produced on cooked foods proves their great systemic resistance. They are using much energy to offset the effects of these foods, and if the system were clean and pure the energy thus consumed might go to enhance the volume and beauty of the voice.

Irritations due to use of voice: Speakers, lecturers, orators, ministers, all are subject to great annoyance when using their voices for a protracted period. A dry irritation, accompanied by a short, rasping cough, will frequently attack them, and they are unable to proceed without the soothing glass of water or lozenge, which relieves them temporarily by lubricating the membranes. If the lubricating glands were functioning properly and they were in a strong, healthy condition, the individuals, would experience no difficulty in talking for hours. The presence of the irritation evinces a disorder of the nasal and respiratory passages. An overstimulation of the lubricating glands produces an excess fluid, which accumulates and clogs the passages, becoming thick and foul-smelling and resulting in what is termed dropping catarrh.

Voice vs. physique: Frequently we find speakers who have puny bodies and deep, resonant voices, whereas a large, well-developed man may have a light voice with little vibration. Again, we find a singer, slight in stature, with a full, flowing voice. Herein lies the explanation. Everyone has more powerful development in some parts of the body than others. Even the chronic invalid has at least one organ which preserves its immunity to a great extent. Some people have powerful stomachs and apparently can digest anything from a Welshrarebit to a tin can, without any subsequent discomfort. Others have vitally strong nervous systems, which withstand shocks, strain and overwork for many years. The small, thin man with the big, booming voice happens to have vigorous respiratory organs, and the greater part of his strength is located in that region, which accounts for his vocal power. The same is true of the singer. Where there is not a perfect co-ordination of all the bodily functions there is not perfect health, and the individual who possesses a voice despite these draw-backs merely has his energy concentrated in those parts of the body from which the voice emanates.

Food the cause of voice troubles: The singers of today think they understand the care of their health. For the most part, they endeavor to cultivate simple tastes and moderate habits and cling to a systematic schedule of living. Indeed, if they did otherwise, their voices would not endure as long as they do. They fail at the outset, though, because they know nothing of foods. With a few exceptions, they eat what they please, and while I do not imply that they all gormandize, I know that the character of their foods is injurious. In spite of their care of themselves, all of our singers are subject to colds and fatigue. Every season we hear of this concert being canceled or that opera postponed because the artist is suffering With a cold. Just recently, before the opera season had even commenced, Garden collapsed after a strenuous and prolonged rehearsal and was under a physician's care for several days. And Mary Garden has an unusually vigorous physical development! What, then, is the reason for the colds, collapses and fatigue which the stars suffer? Food! Food! Food! Demineralized, cooked Food, white sugar, tea, coffee, meat, pastry! Foods which wreck the nerves and destroy the body, produce old age, disease and death.

Singers, speaker lecturers, orators, all of them, lose their hair, their teeth, their eyesight, develop colds, catarrh, influenza, pleurisy, kidney trouble and all the other ills common to the human family. *Do* their voices fortify them against these diseases? Not unless the voice is fortified by health, and health is never built on dead material. We do not plant dead seeds in dead soil to grow live grain or fresh flowers. We do not build houses or furniture of dead wood. If we did, they would soon collapse. Therefore, we cannot build live, healthy bodies on dead food. On the lecture platform, when I have proceeded to this point, I am usually confronted with the hue and cry that our greatest athletes, our keenest literary minds, our great judiciaries and the wizards of finance have been bred on cooked food, because raw foods are a recent innovation. Very well, the athlete's glory is short-lived. He succumbs early. The literary luminaries, the great jurists, as a class, are not high livers. They are generally undernourished types, who burn up their nervous energies and pay small attention to food, and thus escape the early decadence to which their more epicurean brother is susceptible. The man whose brain is in constant action, the writer, creative genius or mechanical inventor, eats enough food to keep him alive, but not enough to bloat and devitalize his body. If he did, his mind would soon lose its brilliancy. The notable financiers are, for the most part, men whose early lives have been fraught with hardship and deprivation, and their progress has been made step by step and with little opportunity for the self-indulgence which is ruinous to health. On the other hand, some of the great figures of commerce have suffered an early collapse by which they profited and after recovery paid scrupulous attention to their health in order to accumulate more millions.

All of these geniuses, regardless of what their specialty may be, are *never* 100% *in everything*. The athlete may be 99% or even 100% in his line, but he seldom attracts attention in any other field. He has forced his development physically and burns out that capacity very early. The great writers, jurists and inventors obtain just enough nourishment and rest to keep their mental activity at a high mark, but do you often find a man in this field who excels in physical development? Rarely. It is my contention that the man who lives on the right kind of food, *Raw Food*, which is live and vital, can build himself to such a high point that his capacity, being so increased, he is able to develop along all lines. Of course, not all men can be writers, athletes and inventors, but it is entirely within the range of possibility for the average man to cultivate more than one talent. He can develop the physical as well as the mental.

No man need be limited to one specialty. We have all heard women complain because their husbands constantly talked shop. These men talk shop because their interests are centered in their one particular line of work. That is justifiable, of course, but if the interests were diversified, the men would possess a broader development and a more interesting personality.   Health means increased energy— a broader capacity.

Brilliant minds, depleted bodies: Edison is an example of the individual whose mind burns like a steady flame, but whose body is devitalized. He prides himself on sleeping but four hours out of 24, and his body is failing rapidly, although he gets just enough rest to feed his brain so that its action is clear and brilliant. Edison's face and body show the need of rest. His muscles droop and sag, his movements are slow, lacking in vigor, showing that the body does not keep pace with the mentality. In striking contrast is Georges Clemenceau, the Tiger of France (he is older than Edison), whose tissues are full and firm, showing rest and nourishment. Clemenceau, realizing the value of sleep, retires early in the evening, around eight o'clock, to insure plenty of rest and relaxation and afford his body ample time to recuperate and build. He is the exception, however, for few people, even physicians, who are supposed to be in possession of the vital facts concerning health but who fail to apply the knowledge, if indeed they really have it, avail themselves of sufficient sleep to fortify their bodies.

Voice teachers limited by lack of knowledge of health. Singers and speakers, professional lecturers, dramatic artists and all others whose occupation or profession involves the constant use of their voice, give small heed to their health and less to their diet and concentrate most of their energy in developing the one talent which they have chosen to follow. Even with their close attention to the technique of voice training there is often some detail overlooked. Few teachers are perfect in all respects and include all points in training a large voice from a thin, poor one. One special-izes in placement; another bends his energies toward coaching and imparting the delicate finish and roundness to the voice. And not even the greatest singers always have perfectly placed voices. Caruso's voice, for the most part, was in his throat. That was discernible, not only in the voice at times but in his position while on the stage. There was usually, accompanying the high tones, a distention of the throat muscles and veins of the face, a general physical strain, as evidenced by the tense, upward lifting of the body as though reaching for a tone, showing the exertion of great bodily effort. I do not mean to cast any reflection on Caruso's voice. I admired it immensely and went to hear him on every possible occasion. I merely cite this to illus-trate what I mean concerning placement. Mura-tore's voice is similarly placed. McCormack possesses that rare thing, a natural correct head placement. Galli-Curci's head tones are the result of studious development, although she and Rosa Raisa are both slight of stature and have not, even now, developed their lungs to the full capacity.

Importance of correct speaking. Every one, aside from speakers and singers, should be taught to speak correctly, and when this is achieved he has at his command the pri-mary rudiments of a singing voice. Ninety-nine people out of a hundred talk in their throats. Their general conversa-tion is a mumble of poorly-articulated words. The lips are used but little, the jaws drop, and the guttural sounds which emanate from the back of the throat but slightly re-semble the original word properly articulated. To speak correctly, the lips and tongue and teeth should be used freely. The tones should strike the sounding board of the head and be brought forward directly on the teeth. Each word should be carefully pronounced, not with affectation, but simply and perfectly, with no omissions or slurring of final letters or syllables. This makes for clean-cut, perfect diction in speaking as well as singing. Cultured, refined people are recognized by their perfect articulation of words and phrases and well-modulated voices, and as one is judged by his speech, it is unnecessary and ill-advised to run the risk of being greatly misjudged for the sake of the few extra seconds required for perfect enunciation and careful placement.

The correct placement of a tone, whether in speaking or singing, has a most important effect upon the health. When the tones are placed in the front part of the head the air passages, the sinuses, the ethmoid and sphenoid bones and the antrum are all oxygenated. The waste accumulations are burned out by the purifying action of the oxygen; the vibrations stimulate all the head cavities and keep them free from poisonous masses. The head and nasal passages are kept open and the dangers of catarrh, polypus and sinus infections are eliminated.

Author's experience. You may ask what knowledge I have of the subject. The answer is, the knowledge which comes with personal experience. Years ago my physical condition was such that I was given up by all my physicians and told that I would live only six months. An inveterate drinker and smoker, I had neglected my health all my life, with the result that I had all the ailments on the calendar, including catarrh and polypus. My head and nose were so clogged that I could scarcely breathe. For years I had treated with nose and throat specialists, but the catarrhal condition advanced to the point where the accumulations dropped into my throat and caused me untold discomfort and embarrassment, as my breath was so offensive I disliked to approach anyone. Finally when I decided to take a new lease on life, I stopped drinking and smoking and began to think about developing my body. After going to bed at eight o'clock every night for a solid year, I built up enough morale and will power to begin in earnest. I realized that if I were to have real health I must thoroughly oxygenate my body, and I decided to develop my lungs by becoming an expert swimmer. It was a slow, difficult process, but I won out by ceaseless effort and close application. I conceived the idea of oxygenating the head to correct the catarrhal conditions, and while I succeeded to a pretty good extent, I was still annoyed with congestion and colds in the head. About this time, my wife was studying vocal music, and, going with her to the studio on several occasions, I determined to take up voice training, not so much for the development of a voice as an accomplishment, but as an aid to health. I realized that through this medium I could develop the glands and cords of my throat and head, improve my speaking voice and general physical condition and in this way obviate disease by increasing my bodily resistance. Accordingly I began, and as my work progressed I realized that, while the various methods employed in development of the voice were reasonably successful, to a great extent, they were more or less haphazard, as each teacher applied his own method to all the voices he trained.   This is an error, as voices, like diseases, require individual diagnosis, and what one voice lacks, another may possess, so that the methods of training have to be adjusted to each particular case. This does not mean that each teacher must have a dozen different methods, but it does mean that to develop a beautiful voice the teacher should be capable of recognizing the needs of each pupil and adapt his methods accordingly. In spite of these shortcomings, however, the voice training, of necessity, forces the singer to use his lungs more than he ever has before, if he is just an average human, and the increased lung capacity means improved health.

Most of the methods of voice training in vogue are far from correct. The average teacher reverses the natural action of the muscles. That is why so many voices are ruined and so few achieve successful development. The rare successes are due to a resistance of the general methods; in other words, the voice is developed in spite of the training and not as a result of it. Instead of correcting my voice I began to lose it and instead of building health I was producing more disease. Upon analyzing the situation, I found that the training was against the natural co-ordination of the muscles. I then began to work out a system of head breathing and studied its application to voice work. The more I studied the action of the muscles of the face and head, the more I realized that the systems were all wrong as far as the production of health simultaneously with voice development was concerned.

The average teacher doesn't look after his own health; in fact, he understands little or nothing about the first principles of health. He may care for himself to the extent of his limited knowledge but his general physical condition is an eloquent testimony of how little he understands or applies the precepts of health. Naturally such people are not qualified to teach health to their pupils. I do not mean to imply that voice teachers should be physical culturists but since the voice is so directly related to the state of health, it is emphatic that the teacher have an understanding of the essentials for building health.

Many pupils take up voice work when they are physically broken down and depleted. The overtaxing of the bodily energy under these conditions is disastrous to both health and voice. The vocal cords and resonator muscles become worn and diseased because the system of training does not permit the air to enter the body in a way to build it. The pupil who is not property instructed in the correct method of breathing, places all the strain upon the throat and vocal cords in order to give the voice power. The forcing of the voice saps the physical energy and destroys the delicate quality of the vocal cords, inflaming and irritating them.

The systems by which an attempt is made to train the voice with the placement in the throat are extremely injurious. There are no resonating chambers in the throat and no voice can vibrate if placed in the throat. Unless the system of breathing is so thoroughly understood that it embraces the entire body, the development of both voice and health is jeopardized. There are some systems which build health from the neck down but not from the neck up. The abdominal, diaphragmatic, intercostal or thoracic breathing advocated by many teachers will strengthen and build those parts of the body which are immediately affected by the breathing but unless a system of *head breathing* is employed, wherein perfect oxygenation of the head clears the passages and cavities, stimulates the circulation and energizes the tissues and membranes, the progress of the voice and health will soon be arrested by the diseased conditions which are the result of clogged and imperfectly oxygenated head areas.

I found that by working *with* Nature instead of against Her that the air passages of the head and throat opened and cleared. The natural method which in no way constricted the muscles but relaxed and made them pliable, worked quickly and effectively. My head cleared and I overcame the stubborn case of catarrh with which I had been long afflicted. The purifying agencies of the oxygen which constantly swept through the head with this system of head breathing, burned out the polypi and other impurities and stimulated the tissues of both head and face.

If one breathes *properly* and *completely,* he develops Health (all things else in proportionate balance, as has been explained in foregoing chapters) and the voice is, of necessity, there, ready to be brought out. Everyone has a voice which is a latent talent. The strength and quality of that voice is in direct proportion to the individual's health and development.

I studied the action of my voice and the reaction of my body until I was thoroughly familiar with the most delicate changes in the voice and could connect them with a previous change in the body. A few nights' loss of sleep, over-exertion, some slight indulgence of seemingly unimportant character, all reflected on the voice in an incredibly brief space of time. These were observations made separately from those of the immediate practice time, such as a poorly-placed tone due to muscular strain or careless diction, etc.

I plodded away, practicing hour after hour, often fatiguing both body and voice purposely, to note the resultant effects and the length of time required for recuperation. With this constant exercise and oxygenation of the head, vocal organs and lungs, the membranes which had been badly inflamed and susceptible to cold and congestion commenced to build and become strong and resistive. The air passages were opened by the constant head breathing and elimination of the poisonous accumulation was effected with plenty of oxygen. Persistence in this work so increased my health that I finally found that I was almost immune from colds. Only when I carelessly allow my energies to be lowered through continued loss of sleep and overwork am I susceptible. I can lose a vast amount of sleep and expend an enormous amount of energy and still hold out against colds for a surprisingly long time, so great is my reserve energy. I am able to lecture for hours without hoarseness or fatigue, water or cough-drops, because I have learned to speak with my lips, tongue, teeth, head passages and throat all coordinating so that not one of them is subjected to the burden of the effort and consequently does not become temporarily exhausted.

Do you think I have succeeded in accomplishing this by living on *cooked foods?* I have *not.* Because to achieve this feat one must have not only perfect co-ordination of the respiratory organs, but great physical power and endurance, and I have yet to see the man who can build endurance and power on *dead* food.

Raw food is the food which builds *power, energy, vitality* and *vigor,* and Raw Food is the only food which will build the kind of a *voice* which will *endure* for years.

THE SUB-CONSCIOUS

The Connecting Link Between the Spirit and the Body

> I teach you Health. You choose your Religion.
>
> *"...and the Father are One."* 1 John X-30.
> *"The Father that dwelleth in me, He doeth the works."* 1 John XIV-10.

When we think a thought, that thought is transmitted to all the cells of the body. Thus they are impelled to act as we wish. If we wish to raise an arm the entire process, from the thought conception to the execution, in Health, is so automatic that apparently both thought and act are simultaneous. Yet the conscious mind is a distinct entity which belongs solely to the physical body. The real incentive for thought and the actual power which impels the vasomotor system of the body after the thought has been flashed to the various nerve centers, is in the Sub-Conscious mind.

When we lie down and go to sleep we are inert and dead, as far as the conscious mind is concerned. The conscious mind has relaxed its action; it has no control over the bodily functions. However, the heart goes on beating, the bloodstream courses through the arteries and veins; the kidneys, liver and spleen continue to function. What is the power which directs this continuous activity of the involuntary organs? It is not the conscious mind, for that controls only the voluntary actions. It is the *sympathetic* nervous system which is controlled by the Sub-Conscious mind.

What is the Sub-Conscious mind? The Sub-Conscious mind is the great Divine force, the God-power within ourselves. The Sub-Conscious is the Divine Intelligence which impregnates the body with the vital elements that give it power, health and development.

The Sub-Conscious is a veritable storehouse of knowledge. It provides the conscious mind with resources for utilization in the conscious body. The conscious mind sows the seeds which grow in the Sub-Conscious. The Sub-Conscious mind never forgets. The impulses, thoughts and desires to which you give expression, though they may not be expressed verbally, are retained in the Sub-Conscious. Thus you find yourself recalling easily, or with effort, as the case may be, ideas which may have occurred to you years ago, dreams which you did not remember for several days or weeks after you had dreamed them, scenes which were visualized for but a fleeting moment. Dates, incidents, names, etc., are automatically filed in the Sub-Conscious mind. If they are of sufficient importance to impress the conscious mind, they are never forgotten by the Sub-Conscious mind, and when the conscious mind has need of them these facts will be yielded over by the Sub-Conscious just as the well-stocked larder provides resources for emergencies of the household.

The sympathetic nervous system is the medium between the Sub-Conscious mind and the physical body. The God force, the Spirit of Life, flows through the sympathetic nervous system, which controls and promotes the action of the involuntary organs. Perfect Health is perfect Harmony, and perfect Harmony is God. If we lack health we lack Harmony and hence we lack the God force. The Spirit of God inhabits us only in proportion to our physical perfections and condition of Health. If we are in perfect Health we manifest God, but we cannot manifest God if our bodies are diseased and our Health broken, for God is Life, and there can be no all-enveloping Life in diseased conditions.

God is not, according to the traditional conception, a Being Who sits in royal state upon a golden throne and administers rewards to the just and punishment to the wicked. God is within ourselves, and we create our own Heaven or Hell.

When we have learned how to live and maintain a state of perfect Health, our minds become clear, keen and active; our bodies are purified, our vibrations are higher and we are brought into closer touch with the universal forces. We acquire the insight and illumination to recognize, understand and use the God-power within ourselves. We live in tune with the Infinite.

Those who pray, and pray and read holy books and attend religious services, but give no heed to their state of health, neglect their bodies and permit them to contract disease and become disordered, are only mentally conceiving the Spirit of God. They are not experiencing the benefits which may be derived from the use of the God power inside themselves. They have only a mental picture of the Divinity. Their bodies are battered and broken, and God does not dwell in ruined temples. As there can be no sanctity in an unholy place, neither can there be any spirituality in a diseased body. There may be the mental desire for spirituality, but it cannot be ideally developed without the co-ordination and harmony of the physical body.

When the body is strong and vibrant, the mind is keen and the thoughts come freely and clearly; the spirit is predominant. Thoughts are living things which can be photographed. This is an impressive fact, the contemplation of which should induce a resolve to guard our thoughts and control them that they may be worthy ones and not the idle, shallow products of an undisciplined mind. When the body is assailed by disease the strength is depleted, the mind becomes sluggish, the thoughts then are slow in forming, and hazy and indefinite, proving that the Spirit power is diminished and God does not inhabit His temple.

This great Sub-Conscious force within us governs our every action. It supplies the motive for our conscious actions, and it controls our involuntary actions. When we are relaxed and sleeping, if this Sub-Conscious power stops, if God takes leave of his tabernacle, we die at once. The life forces cease to flow into the sympathetic nervous system, which is the medium between the Sub-Conscious and the physical body, and the heart stops beating. This brings us to the realization that the Creator dwells directly within us. When our bodies become diseased and broken, they are finally condemned to die. The Spirit withdraws then, as we vacate a condemned house or building because it is no longer worthy to dwell in.

The Sub-Conscious is one of the Trinity, God's composite creation, the Spiritual, Mental and Physical. There is no separation as so many people think. God is within us, we are made in His image and likeness, and only when we defile that likeness by filling it with impurities is the Spirit driven from it.

When you become fully acquainted with the fact that God dwells within you, that you are one and there is no separation, then you will be able to fulfill your mission on earth.

The great trouble is that all teachings concerning the Divinity have to do with the mental only, with no thought for the physical. Divine Harmony is attained only through perfect co-ordination of the Trinity—Spiritual, Mental and Physical. When sickness and disease oppress us we have transgressed against the Laws of God. We are out of Harmony with the Divine. The physical then lacks proper adjustment and the influences which permit the Superior Intelligence to guide it.

We have no power of our own. All power comes to us through the Divinity, Who works within us, and the more completely we comprehend this and perfect our physical bodies, the more expansive will be our development and government by the God within ourselves. Our brain power, physical strength and spiritual comprehension will be unlimited, because we shall be uniting all of the forces at our command and achieving perfect equalization.

For centuries we have groped blindly for the secret of Life, seeking God, when all along the true and living God has dwelt within our bodies, overlooked, neglected and unheeded.

God is Good; God is Love; God is All in All. God is Health; therefore to express God perfectly your body must be in a state of Health. Get in touch with God by building your body to use its fullest powers. Become a superman or superwoman.

The Sub-Conscious is the Spirit force which rules you at all times, asleep or awake. To receive the full Power of the Sub-Conscious it is essential that the body be kept healthy and vital so that the Spirit forces may flow into the medium through which they control the body, namely, the sympathetic nervous system.

And now you ask, "What has all of this to do with raw foods?" Answer: *It is the link in the chain* that connects the *Divine* and *Spirit force* with tithe body, namely: the raw food is the food designed by God to keep perfect His image and I likeness. It is God's command that you should live on the fruits, herbs and seeds in the state He grew them, 100% for a 100% body.

Now let us analyze it and see if it is so. The life of the cooked food is destroyed in cooking, robbed of its vitamins and of its energy. Where there was 100% before being cooked, it has now lost from 40 to 90 per cent of its nutritional value by being cooked. The energy you receive in this small amount of nutrition is not sufficient to carry off the poisons produced by the waste of the meal you have just eaten.

When the poisons from this meal are partially eliminated, your nerves cry out for the minerals they need to produce health, which can only be supplied in the raw food. Not having the necessary amount of these in the cooked foods, you slowly become diseased. In other words, you lack the live minerals in your food to attract the Life force, which is Spiritual, to your body, which is physical.

Have you ever asked yourself how the Life —or God-force, is attracted to your body? The raw food, cereals, vegetables, fruits and nuts are 100% nourishment in their natural state and contain the same minerals that the body is made up of. When you consume these in their natural state they produce health through their power of being alive. These live minerals bring about a chemical, an electro-magnetic change in the body, that attracts and draws unto itself (the physical body) the Spirit Power, or God-force, through the Sub-Conscious into the sympathetic nervous system and through this involuntary process the Spirit of Life force is transmitted to all of the involuntary organs, and then in turn to the conscious mind and the voluntary parts of the body, there to be used for constructive or destructive action, according to the impressions of the conscious mind. Reason this out for yourself and ask yourself if cooked food, which is dead and robbed of its life-producing minerals, or anything else that is a corpse, has the power to attract *anything* unto itself, much less *Life.*

There is no chance for an argument here except with a diseased and unbalanced mind. Those of you who have not known how to express God as He wished you to in His name and likeness, which is Health, and are satisfied to pray and waste His time reading the Bible with a blank mind and not trying to understand Him and analyze His beautiful and natural teachings, draw on your mental force and analyze His following words and see if you are living according to His teachings or not:

**"And God said, Behold, I have given
you every herb bearing seed which is
upon the face of all the earth, and every**

tree, in the which is the fruit of a tree yielding seed; to you it shall be for meat.

"And to every beast of the earth, and to every fowl of the air, and to everything that creepeth upon the earth, wherein there is life, I have given every green herb for meat; and it was so"— *Genesis* 1-29-30.

Purify the body by fasting. Build it and keep it in perfect health by eating God's foods in their natural raw state. The physical will then vibrate Life, Energy and Power, which constitute perfect Health. God will then inhabit His temple and yours will be a long and blessed life free from disease.

Foods and Menus

INTRODUCTORY

"To spoil it—boil it."

The following menus and suggestions have been made up with the intent to simplify the preparation of meals as much as possible. It is my contention that the hours which have previously been spent in the elaborate preparation of unhealthful meals may now be used in the more profitable way of developing the mind and body. The simpler a meal, the more beneficial it is. Even with uncooked food it is not wise to combine more than two or three vegetables, and they must not be taken in excess. The raw foods carry so much nourishment—they are 100%—that discretion must be exercised lest the stomach be overloaded. As you become accustomed to the uncooked diet, you will find that you are easily satisfied with a smaller amount of food. Where you used to require at least three courses—meat, salad and dessert, or soup, meat and dessert —you will find your appetite gratified with a salad and some milk.

I do not advocate ground and crushed vegetables to any extent. Only in cases where the teeth are gone and artificial ones have replaced them or where the teeth and gums are extremely sensitive, due to pyorrhea conditions and general neglect, and in cases of young children whose teeth are not fully developed, should it be necessary to

macerate the food. In these cases, of course, it would be difficult to eat the raw vegetables, so I recommend that the
vegetable be ground and the nuts flaked in order to accommodate the food to the tender mouths. At all times the
food must be thoroughly masticated. This applies to those
who have teeth and those who haven't. The people who
have teeth can keep them longer by giving them sturdy
use. Nothing so strengthens the jaws and muscles of the
face and prolongs the life of the teeth as thorough mastication of firm foods. The tissues of the mouth are stimulated
and new circulation carried to the teeth. You may ask why
it is necessary for anyone without teeth to masticate his
food. *Because thorough insalivation of food is essential to perfect
assimilation.* The longer food is chewed the more perfectly
the saliva is blended with it, and when it enters the stomach it is ready for the digestive process and eventual
assimilation. The stomach was not intended to do the
teeth's work, and although in most cases it makes a brave
attempt, the results are most unsatisfactory. All food should
be chewed so thoroughly that it becomes a creamy liquid in
the mouth. When you take a mouthful of food, chew that
mouthful thoroughly without swallowing any part of it. If
you have an uncontrollable impulse to swallow, then swallow muscularly but do not permit any of the food to slip
down the throat. When you have masticated your food to
the proper creamy consistency, it will flow down the throat
with the action of the mastication.

MENUS

Twenty Centuries ago Seneca, the Roman philosopher, said: "Man does not die—he kills himself."

Breakfast

I.
Cantaloupe
Whole Wheat Bread with
Butter and Honey
Glass of Milk

II.
Egg whipped to froth
flavored with Lemon Juice
and Honey
Glass of Milk

III.
Large glass of Orange Juice

IV.
Sliced Bananas and Raisins
Whole Grain sprinkled over top
Cream may be used

V.
Chopped Figs and Whole Grain with Cream

VI.
Three glasses of Milk and Cream

VII.
Berries without Cream or Sugar Whole
Wheat Bread, toasted or plain

VIII.
Fresh sliced Pineapple

IX.
Raisins with Cream

X.
Choice of White Grapes Tokay Grapes
Malaga Grapes

A breakfast may be made entirely on fruit juice or the fruits themselves. If acid fruit is taken, drink no milk and eat no bread. (Cooked starch should not be taken with *acid* fruits.)

Do not eat too many eggs. They carry a large amount of protein, and unless you are using a great deal of physical energy they have a tendency to make you bilious and heavy.

Canned fruits should not be used. They carry white sugar and preservatives.

Luncheons and Dinners
Eat Wisely, but not too well.

I.

Lettuce and Pineapple Salad Cream or
Pimento Cheese

II.

Tomato stuffed with Chopped Celery
Garnished with Lettuce
Mayonnaise Dressing Honey

III.

Cottage Cheese with Finely-chopped
Green Peppers and Onions
Milk or Cream
(This may be served with lettuce as a salad or
made into thin Sandwiches)

IV.

Fresh Spinach Leaves Raw Cauliflower
Shredded Beets
(Use Spinach same as Lettuce)
Milk or Cream

V.

Head Lettuce Diced or Grated Carrots
Chopped Onions, with Sprinkling of

Raw Peanuts
Serve with Mayonnaise or French Dressing
(Use Lemon Juice instead of Vinegar)
Milk or Cream

VI.
Dates stuffed with Cream or Cottage Cheese
Serve on Lettuce with Mayonnaise
Dressing Milk or Cream

VII.
Head Lettuce Serve with French Dressing to
which has been added the pulp of a large Tomato,
a table-spoonful each of Chopped Cucumbers
and Onions
(This makes an attractive, palatable salad)
Garnish with Sliced Radishes

VIII.
Celery stuffed with Pimento or Cream Cheese
Diced Young Turnips
Whole Wheat Bread
Milk or Cream

IX.
Tomato stuffed with Shredded Cabbage
Mayonnaise or French Dressing
Radishes Onions
Milk or Cream

X.
Young Corn on Cob
Salad of Lettuce, Water Cress or
Endive Milk

XL
Green Peas and Beans
(Put through vegetable grinder)
Serve on Lettuce with Mayonnaise or French
Dressing or Use to stuff Tomato
Milk or Cream

XII.
Young Asparagus Tips
Serve on Lettuce with Mayonnaise or French
Dressing or in combination with other vegetables

Carbohydrates

Raisins	Figs
Prunes	Dates

Proteins

Eggs	Milk
Cheese	Nuts

Acids

Rhubarb	Lemons
Grapefruit	Oranges

Non-Starchy Vegetables

Celery	Tomatoes
Cabbage	Cucumbers
Spinach	Radishes
Kale	Onions
Watercress	

Semi-Acids

Grapes	Peaches
Sweet Oranges	Pears
Apples	

It is not necessary that each meal contain some of the types of food mentioned above, but to give the system what it requires and maintain a balance it is necessary to eat some of all of the elements which form the composition of the body.

SOUPS

Because most soups have to be cooked to be palatable, their use is limited by people who wish to live on a diet of raw foods.

As a substitute for soups, in arranging a meal, the fruit cocktails or punches may be used.

It is, of course, always advisable to eat the fruits in their natural state. For aged people and infants who have no teeth and invalids who are not allowed solid foods, the juices may be extracted from the fruit and administered instead of broths and soups. All cooked soups are 99 per cent water and their nutritive values negligible. Fruit juices substituted are cleansing, stimulating and nourishing and have important medicinal properties.

SOUPS (Remarks)

Grain stock for cream soups can be made by soaking one or more kinds of grain together until soft enough to put through a ricer, making a creamy mass, to which milk and seasoning can be added.

Fresh vegetable can be made from the juice of tomatoes, to which can be added chopped vegetables and seasoning.

Fruit soups are: made by extracting the juice from any juicy fruit and adding water, honey and sometimes a little lemon juice or other fruit macerated.

If a warm soup is desired in winter it may be slightly heated and served in rather heavy bowls which have previously been heated.

A few suggestions for above soups:

Cream of Corn. Soak overnight or until soft enough about one-half pound of grain (either one or more kinds together) and put through ricer. Add enough milk to desired thickness. Then shred or mash some corn, peas, celery or other vegetable desired and season with powdered celery, sage or other seasoning and add grated onion juice if desired.

Vegetable Soup. Put the pulp and seeds of six large tomatoes through a strainer and add chopped parsley, grated onion or onion juice. Any chopped or grated vegetable may be added to this, together with a very small amount of something of a pronounced flavor, such as parsnips or horseradish. Then season to taste.

Fruit Soup. To 1 pint of pure grape juice add 1 cup of water, the juice of half a lemon and enough honey to sweeten to taste. To this may be added a banana finely macerated. Pineapple or other fruits and berries may be added to give more flavor if desired. Shredded mint leaves may be added.

These are only suggestions, from which the housewife can make any variety she wishes.

SALADS

Every day you poison a divine spirit, body,
mind, youth and energy by the dead,
cooked food you eat.

Vegetables to be used in salads: Lettuce, spinach, carrots, celery, radishes, onions, cucumbers, tomatoes, sweet and Irish potatoes, red, white and curly cabbage, parsnips, endive, chicory, kale, chard, chives, beans, peas, beets, oyster plant, white and yellow turnips, egg-plant, carrots, leeks, parsley, horseradish, celery roots, pumpkin, squash—in fact, anything that grows as a vegetable can be used in salads.

Vegetables which cannot be eaten whole or sliced, such as beets, carrots, turnips, etc., can be chopped fine or shredded.

Young tender cauliflower can be used by breaking in a few pieces into the salad or chopping it fine.

Young asparagus tips may be used whole in the salad or sliced in very thin slices.

Green or wax beans may be used in salads by slicing very fine crosswise.

Dried beans, peas, lima beans, etc., can be used in salad by soaking until soft enough to put through vegetable grinder and sprinkled over salad.

Any leafy vegetable can be used as a base for salad, as lettuce, spinach, water cress, chard, endive, etc., using two or more other vegetables in combination.

SALADS
Vegetable Combinations

Lettuce, tomatoes, cucumbers and onions. Lettuce, cauliflower, peas and carrots. Lettuce, green pepper and asparagus tips. Lettuce, cabbage and celery.

Lettuce, beet and celery.
Lettuce, tomatoes and green peas.

Lettuce, green pepper, celery and beans.
Lettuce, brussels sprouts and chicory.
Lettuce, celery and radishes.
Lettuce, cabbage and carrots.
Water cress, cauliflower and beet.
Water cress, cucumber and tomato.
Spinach and cauliflower.
Swiss chard, tomato and onion.
Kale, celery and green peppers.
Kale, beet and celery.
Lettuce, celery and apple.
Lettuce, dates and nuts.
Spinach, cottage cheese.
Spinach, apple, celery and nut.
Lettuce, prunes and nuts.
Spinach,   banana, cocoanut and grated carrot.
Lettuce, banana, flaked peanuts.

SALADS
Fruit Combinations

Lettuce, strawberries, pineapple, oranges
    and bananas.

Lettuce, oranges and bananas.
Lettuce, oranges and prunes.
Lettuce, apples, bananas and pineapples.
Spinach, dates, oranges and pineapples.
Spinach, peaches, bananas and grapes.
Spinach, pineapples, figs and oranges.
Spinach, pineapple, prunes and peaches.
Water cress, bananas, grapes and figs.
Water cress, pineapple and cocoanut.
Water cress and avocado pear.
Water cress, dates and nuts.
Endive, pineapple and cream cheese.

DECORATIVE SALADS

Filled Apples. Scoop out the centers of nice red apples. Mix with the apples that have been scooped out chopped celery and walnuts and mayonnaise dressing. Fill shells with this mixture and put a teaspoonful of whipped cream on top of each. Serve on lettuce leaves.

Filled Peppers. Fill pimentos or sweet peppers with following mixture: Rub cream or cottage cheese to a paste with a little cream. Add grated onion, chopped nuts and shredded beets. Serve on lettuce or spinach.

Filled Cabbage. Serve in tender cabbage leaf the mixture of finely-chopped cabbage, celery and onion. Add to this one cup of chopped nuts. Mix all together with equal parts of lemon juice and olive oil.

Red Cabbage Salad. To one cream cheese add one finely-chopped sweet pepper; add one cup chopped celery and two cups new red cabbage, finely chopped; moisten with a little cream and serve on tender white cabbage leaves.

Cheese and Tomato Salad. Cut large, smooth tomatoes into six sections, not severing the sections and allow to fall open like a flower. Mix: cream cheese with paprika and grated onion. Put mixture through potato ricer and fill each center. Serve on lettuce or spinach leaves.

Date and Cheese Salad. Remove stones from required amount of dates and fill with cream cheese. Arrange in bed of lettuce and serve with French dressing. Prunes may be served in the same way.

Cucumber and Nut Salad. Cut a cucumber in half. Remove seeds and fill hollow with chopped nuts mixed with grated cheese Sprinkle with chopped parsley and serve on water cress or endive.

Raw Food Salad. Put through fine vegetable grinder one stalk celery, one sweet potato, one carrot, one apple, one small yellow turnip, one beet, one cup seeded raisins, one cup walnuts and pecans. Put into this one cup of olive oil and let stand for several hours. When ready to serve add the juice of two lemons. Serve on young spinach leaves or lettuce.

Grape Fruit Salad. To shredded grape fruit add chopped celery, apples, bananas, figs and dates. Mix with mayonnaise or French dressing and serve in grape fruit shells lined with tender lettuce leaves.

Mock Lobster Salad. To grated carrots add a little grated horseradish. Mix with half the quantity of chopped celery and nuts. Place lettuce hearts on a platter and arrange carrot mixture in center of each to resemble the shape of a lobster as nearly as possible. Serve with mayonnaise and slices of lemon.

Nasturtium Salad. On a bed of tender nasturtium leaves, slice a layer of tomatoes, then a layer of sliced cucumbers and on top of this young sweet corn cut from the cob. Serve with French dressing and garnish with nasturtium flowers.

(Lindlahr.)

Stuffed Tomato Salad. Scoop out tomato and fill with pulp to which has been added chopped cabbage, celery, apples and nuts. Garnish with green peppers.

Orange Basket. Cut orange into shape of a basket forming handle in center. Remove the inside. Fill basket with sliced bananas, pieces of orange, grapes (seeded), chopped dates and nuts. Before serving, place a spoonful of whipped cream on top. Serve on plate with something green to garnish.

Avocado Pear Salad. Cut pears in half. Remove center and serve with French dressing. Serve on endive.

Stuffed Celery Salad. Choose large tender celery stalks; wash and dry and fill hollows with following mixture: one cream cheese rubbed to paste with a little cream and with paprika and onion juice.

Cantaloupe Salad. Peel cantaloupe, remove seeds; and cut into dice. Serve with mayonnaise; or French dressing.

SALAD DRESSINGS

Mayonnaise. To the well beaten yolks of two eggs add one-quarter teaspoon of dry mustard, one-half teaspoon of honey. Mix until well blended. Then add one cup olive oil slowly and juice of one lemon, alternating oil and lemon juice.

French Dressing. To one teaspoon of honey add a dash of paprika. Mix well and add slowly one cup olive oil and the juice of one lemon, alternating oil and lemon juice.

Cream Dressing. To the juice of one lemon add one tablespoon each of onion juice and olive oil. Then slowly add one cup of beaten cream.

Nut Butter Dressing. To one part of lemon juice add two parts of peanut butter. Sweeten to taste.

Estes Special Dressing. To one cup of French dressing add, finely chopped, one small onion, two or three radishes, one small cucumber and pulp of a tomato, one pepper, green or red, enough celery for flavor. Mix all together and use on any vegetable salad.

Mix with mayonnaise dressing for variety, chopped onion, green pepper, grated carrots or beets.

SANDWICHES

Sandwiches of whole wheat or whole rye bread with various fillings, such as cheese of all varieties or prepared in the following manner are delicious:

Finely-cut celery, with or without dressing, on lettuce.

To one cream cheese, add one pimento finely macerated and add a little cream.

Cream or Neufchatel cheese with minced onion, chopped nuts, parsley or green pepper.

Combination Sandwich: Lettuce with sliced tomato, minced onion and mayonnaise.

Dates or figs chopped and mixed with cream cheese.

Cottage cheese with minced onion and green pepper.

Lettuce with mayonnaise.

Finely-chopped nuts with mayonnaise on lettuce.

Chopped onions, nuts and green pepper with mayonnaise.

Peanut butter with chopped raisins and nuts.

Nuts, sundried olives and onions chopped fine and mixed with mayonnaise.

Water cress with mayonnaise.

Cranberries, macerated and sweetened with honey.

Chopped nuts may be sprinkled over any salad. In fact, nuts should be eaten daily in the salad or in some form.

Dried fruits, if sun-dried soaked overnight in just enough water to cover, are delicious used in salads in winter if fresh fruits cannot be had.

Corn, when young and fresh, is delicious eaten from the cob. When not young enough to eat that way, the kernels can be slit down the cob with a sharp knife and the inner part scraped out.

Vegetables, such as carrots, beets, turnips, squash, parsnips, etc., can be chopped for salad, put through vegetable grinder or shredded on Gilmore's coarse or fine shredders. (Apples with skins on are delicious shredded on coarse shredder.) Skins should never be removed from either fruit or vegetables.

DESSERTS AND SAUCES

Prune Whip. Remove pits from one pound of prunes that have been soaked until very soft. Strain through colander and add the stiffly-beaten white of one egg. Cover top with whipped cream, sprinkle with nuts.

Banana Whip. Macerate and whip three ripe bananas. Add a few drops of lemon juice and sweeten with honey. Before serving, add the stiffly-beaten white of one egg.

Fruit and Nut Combination. Cut into small pieces (enough for three layers) grapes, oranges, figs and fresh grated pineapple. Arrange in layers and sprinkle fresh grated coconut between each layer. Slice bananas on top and cover with cocoanut.

Date Cream. To one pint of whipped cream add one cup of chopped dates. Sprinkle top with chopped nuts. Figs may be used instead of dates.

Fruit Mixture. To one pint of stiffly-beaten cream add a little honey to sweeten. Fold in lightly one cup of strawberries cut in halves, one cup shredded pineapple, one banana and one orange cut into small pieces. Sprinkle over with nuts.

Candy. Chop or grind one cup of nut meats, one cup figs, one-half cup dates. Add one tablespoon of orange juice and one square of unsweetened chocolate. Roll out on board, sprinkle with nuts and cut into shapes.

Honey Dessert. To two parts of finely chopped nuts add one part of honey. Mix thoroughly. Cover with whipped cream and stiffly-beaten white of egg.

Uncooked Fruit Cake. Place on a small dish a layer of ground figs and over this a layer of grated nuts and dates cut into small pieces. Cover with fresh grated coconut. Build these layers until of desired thickness. Cover top with fresh cocoanut. Cut thin with sharp knife and serve in small portions.

(Christian.)

ICE CREAM AND ICES

Ice Cream (Plain). Four eggs well beaten. Add to this one cup of honey and slowly beat into this one quart of whipped cream, vanilla flavor. This can be used plain or any kind of crushed fruit added to it just before putting into freezer. Half milk may also be substituted for cream.

Maple Ice Cream. To one pint of whipped cream add one pint of pure maple syrup. Whip until thick. Then add the beaten whites of two eggs and one cupful chopped nuts.

Strawberry Ice. Sweeten with honey three pints of crushed berries. Let this stand to blend about one-half hour. Then add three pints of water and freeze.

Strawberry Sherbet. Put one quart of strawberries through the strainer. Then add the juice of one lemon and sweeten with honey. Put in freezer and when about half frozen add the stiffly-beaten whites of two eggs.

Pineapple Sherbet. To one grated fresh pineapple add enough water to make a quart. Sweeten with honey and freeze. When nearly frozen add the beaten whites of two eggs.

Raspberry Ice. To three cups of fresh raspberry juice add the juice of two lemons and four cups of water. Sweeten to taste with honey and allow it to stand one-half hour to blend. Then put into freezer, and when about half frozen add one-half pint of whipped cream.

Peach Sherbet. Strain one quart of ripe peaches through a strainer. Sweeten with honey and add one cup water and four beaten egg whites and freeze. Other fruits may be substituted for peaches.

Note: As the different varieties of honey are not alike in sweetness, it must be left to the individual to sweeten to taste.

DRINKS

Lemonade. Made in the usual way. Sweeten with honey instead of sugar.

Orangeade. To the juice of eight oranges add the juice of three lemons. Sweeten to taste with honey and add water. Garnish with mint leaves.

Rhubarbcade. Sweeten one-half pint rhubarb juice with honey and add water.

Grapeade. To one quart of grape juice add the juice of six lemons. Sweeten to taste with honey and add water.

Pineappleade. To the juice of one medium sized pineapple add the juice of five lemons and three pints of water. Sweeten to taste with honey.

Mintade. To one handful of crushed mint leaves add the juice of six lemons. Sweeten with honey and let stand one-half hour. Before serving add one-half grape juice and one-half water.

CHEESE

All cheese is cooked and heavily salted. It has its nutritive merits, but because it is constipating and heavy and not in harmony with perfect metabolism of the body, it should be avoided.

The exception is home-made, unsalted cottage cheese, which can be made without cooking. The sour milk is barely heated, just enough to cause it to congeal. It is then poured into a cloth and allowed to drain.

Used in salads, sandwiches, mixed with honey or chopped peppers and onions, it forms a satisfying meal and is highly beneficial.

Remarks. Cottage cheese can be served in many ways, by adding chopped onion, green peppers, pimentos, parsley, cucumbers, radishes or chives, and served to the family once or twice a week. Served on lettuce leaves, it makes a splendid salad. Honey may be added if desired.

Soft cream cheese can be mixed with nuts or figs and used as a stuffing for dates or prunes; or rolled into balls and dipped in chopped nuts it is appetizing with any fruit or vegetable salad.

Grind one-half pound figs and mix thoroughly with one cake of cream cheese.

This may be made mixed with dates as well.

EGGS

Eggs have great nutritious value, but they are capable of causing many digestive disorders if eaten too freely.

In cases of mal-nutrition, extreme depletion and weakness, as tuberculosis, convalescence from typhoid, influenza, etc., raw eggs beaten and mixed with milk, or raw eggs beaten and combined with lemon juice and sweetened with honey, nourish and build the body and restore the strength.

Eggs should be eaten raw and never to excess.

The regular eating of eggs overworks the liver, produces gas, constipation and an excess of albuminous matter in the system. The kidneys are apt to become involved and general complications set up.

Due to the sulphurous matter contained in eggs, they are apt to cause skin disorders if indiscriminately eaten.

Remarks: A refreshing way to eat raw egg is to beat one egg well and add a few drops of lemon juice and one teaspoon of honey.

Eggnog. One egg, well beaten, one cup milk, one teaspoon honey. Beat all together and sprinkle top with nutmeg. Flavor with vanilla.

Maple-egg. One egg well beaten, one cup milk, one tablespoon maple syrup. Beat all together and top with nutmeg or cinnamon.

FRUIT JUICES

The curative and building agencies of orange and lemon juices are almost *unparalleled*. Because the juices of the citric fruits are more easily extracted they have a wider and more practical use. They deposit an alkaline ash in the body which absorbs the acid wastes.

They cleanse, stimulate and nourish the body, reduce adipose tissue and supply the system with the necessary mineral salts.

Grape, blackberry, cherry and blueberry juice are all valuable blood and nerve tonics. They contain large percentages of potassium and iron.

ORANGES

The wonderful effects and nourishment of the orange is almost beyond comparison in its general uses for clearing out the body, stimulating nerve action and overcoming ills. It should be universally used by every household much more than it is. In my treatments for chronic head and tooth troubles and general nerve building (which are done through fasting) I have never found anything so beneficial. Everyone should eat more oranges.

LEMON JUICE

Lemon juice is a simple effective remedy for many disorders, but its curative agencies are overlooked and unappreciated.

Skin eruptions and wounds. Undiluted lemon juice applied to external ulcers, pimples, wounds, and boils has an extraordinarily healing effect. The lemon juice should be allowed to dry on the affected part. It forms a varnish-like coat and the part should not be bandaged, but left exposed to the air.

Eyes. Bathe the eyes with equal parts of tepid water and lemon juice. It allays local inflammation of the eyes. If it has a tendency to sting and burn, the strength of the solution should be modified.

Catarrh. Equal parts of lemon juice and tepid water. The solution in small quantities should be poured into the nostrils with a spoon. With the head tipped back and to one side the liquid will trickle through the nostrils. Treat each nostril in turn.

Long-standing and stubborn cases of catarrh have been promptly relieved by this simple remedy.

Catarrh in all forms is an ailment which is not regarded seriously enough. It has been proved that nasal catarrh is often the forerunner of consumption. The complications which result from neglect of catarrhal conditions in the Head, stomach and intestines are serious and often fatal.

Ear troubles. Use lemon juice and warm water same as for catarrh. Most frequently inner-ear troubles are the result of inflamed Eustachian tubes, which lead from the mouth to the ear. A few drops of warm, undiluted lemon juice in the ear will relieve ear-ache.

Colds, sore throat, bronchitis and asthma. Take a few drops of pure lemon juice on a spoon, open the mouth and toss the juice to the back of the throat. Repeat frequently. This treatment will be found useful to singers and speakers. The source of trouble in these cases is usually in the nasal passages above the throat, so gargling is ineffective. Sipping dilutes the lemon juice and weakens its strength.

Gastric troubles with infants or children. Give a teaspoonful of undiluted lemon juice without sugar every half hour. It allays the stomach irritation, checks vomiting and has a general curative effect The juices of citric fruits have an *alkaline* reaction in the system and will not produce a *hyper-acidic* condition in the body, as many people suppose.

The juice of half a lemon in a cup of cold water taken upon arising in the morning will have a favorable reaction on the liver and skin. People who have muddy, sallow complexions will find this treatment an aid to beauty as well as health.

BUTTERMILK

Buttermilk has a valuable medicinal effect on the body. It destroys the colonic bacteria, absorbs the acid wastes of the body which cause so much disease, corrects digestive disorders and is highly nutritious.

Because of the high percentage of protein the body carries, it can be used with great success in reducing the excess weight of people whose bodies are bloated with retained poisons and un-eliminated waste. On a diet of buttermilk alone adipose tissue can be destroyed, the poisons eliminated and the weight restored to normal without the patients losing strength or looking hollow-eyed and emaciated. The nutritive properties of the buttermilk build the body and augment the strength while the reducing process is going on.

In cases where the body is surcharged with poisons resulting from acidosis, irritability, functional and organic disorders, etc., the medicinal merits of buttermilk cannot be too highly emphasized. It is a corrective of general nervous diseases, for if the system is thoroughly cleansed by fasting, followed by a buttermilk diet, the nerves are properly nourished and built up and their tendencies to disease obviated.

A buttermilk diet should follow a short fast. If the buttermilk is used in conjunction with a plentiful supply of drinking water and acid fruits, the effects will be very gratifying.

The water, buttermilk and fruits should be taken on a schedule at alternate hours of the day, arranging it so the buttermilk is due about the time food is ordinarily taken, thus acting as a substitute for the usual meal. By alternating the three foods, none becomes distasteful and each one has its distinctive effects on the body.

GRAINS

Wheat, rye, barley, corn, oats, rice and millet. These grains are most commonly used.

Grains can be eaten by soaking over night, either one kind or two or three in combination. If the teeth are in a condition where the whole kernel cannot be thoroughly masticated, the grain can be coarsely ground and eaten for breakfast, together with raisins, figs, dates or bananas, or sprinkled over fresh fruit. Dried fruits can be used in winter after having been soaked overnight.

If sweetening is desired, always use honey. Cream may also be added to these breakfast dishes.

LEGUMES

Legumes, such as dried peas, navy beans, lima beans and lentils, may be soaked overnight and put through vegetable grinder and sprinkled over a salad.

BREAD AND WHOLE GRAINS

The use of bread dates centuries back, before Biblical times. It has always been regarded as a most essential part of a meal. Because it has been universally used, it has become a habit with most people, who eat it mechanically.

Because of cooked starches contained in it and their tendency to produce gas and fermentation, I do not advocate bread, but the whole grains instead. In manufacturing most flour, the husks, or outer coats, are removed from the grain and the starchy parts of the grain are crushed up into the flour from which the bread is made. Thus the most valuable part of the grain is destroyed, for the outer coverings contain the essential minerals and vita-mines.

This is particularly true of white flour. Many brands of whole rye, whole wheat and bran flour and bread are on the market but it is more healthful to eat the whole grains themselves instead of the demineralized patent flours.

All the nourishment is retained in the whole grains, which may be soaked overnight and eaten as a cereal with cream and honey or in combination with fruits. Unpolished rice, whole wheat and oats and even barley make very palatable substitutes for bread. They retain a certain firmness even after they have been soaked to facilitate mastication. This resistance to mastication stimulates the teeth and the thorough chewing necessitated by their use increases; the flow of the digestive juices and aids assimilation.

Many cases of distention, dyspepsia and constipation are due to the inordinate consumption of the cooked starches contained in bread, potatoes, beans and polished rice.

Unlike cooked starches, the raw starches do not ferment. The body absorbs what it requires and the remainder is eliminated. No bloating, flatulence or discomfort follows the eating of the raw whole grains.

FRUITS AND NUTS

All fruits are nutritious. Some carry proteins. Others possess the mineral elements which most bodies greatly lack. Bananas, grapes, dates, figs and raisins are highly nourishing and building, and constitute a meal in themselves. Grapes are particularly lauded for their great building properties. Undernourished and greatly fatigued people can increase their weight and strength by eating grapes plentifully when they are in season. They contain a great deal of sugar and create energy and heat in the body. Bananas are rich in proteins and therefore very nourishing but should be eaten with discretion as they are heavy and apt to cause constipation unless they are thoroughly masticated and insalivated. Dates and figs are important nutritive fruits and have a desirable laxative effect. Raisins are blood builders. They contain iron in its most assimilable form and should form an important part of every one's diet.

Great care should be exercised in the selection of figs, dates and raisins as the appetizing products exhibited for sale are generally bleached and preserved by artificial methods. This is particularly true of dates and figs, and raisins are included. To render them more attractive in appearance, they are subjected to a sulphur bleaching process which drains out the natural sugar. To restore the sweet flavor, the fruits are then treated with glycerine which is a coal-tar by-product and very injurious to the human body.

Natural sun-dried fruits are black and wrinkled and resemble a prune. What they lack in appearance they make up for in flavor and nutritional value. Figs that are moist and sticky and raisins which are light in color (except the raisins made from white grapes) have all been artificially treated. Avoid using them.

Apples, oranges, pears, cherries, grapes, peaches, etc., should be eaten with their skins on. Exercise the teeth by chewing the skins thoroughly and extract all of their nutritive and medicinal properties.

Nuts. Nuts contain the protein which is essential to the body. Nuts are highly nutritious and a small quantity eaten with fruits constitutes a well-balanced and thoroughly satisfying meal. No one can live on fruits and vegetables alone. On such a restricted diet, the body would receive only the mineral salts and no proteins. Nuts supply the protein and should be eaten frequently, but not in large quantities. Thorough mastication is absolutely essential to insure perfect digestion and assimilation. Nut and fruit, and nut and vegetable combinations are appetizing and nourishing.

HONEY

Honey is a concentrated natural sweet which should be used instead of sugar and wherever sugar is ordinarily used.

Honey belongs to the carbohydrate group of foods. It creates heat, power and energy in the body. It should be given children as a substitute for candy. Honey gratifies the craving for sweet and builds the body, while the acid-producing white sugar in candy wrecks the digestive processes and depletes the nerve vitality.

It has been observed that people who ate a great deal of honey escaped such contagious diseases as measles, smallpox and scarlet fever when they were very directly exposed to the diseases while those about them who did not eat honey, contracted the diseases to which they were exposed.

VINEGAR

Vinegar is a poison. It is acetic acid and its action on the stomach membranes is highly detrimental. Vinegar dries and destroys the mucous secretions of the stomach. It causes acidosis and biliousness. It tightens and constricts the tissues and dries the skin.

The bacterial condition of the teeth is produced by the acid secretions of the body. If the natural alkalinity is destroyed by vinegar, the secretions become highly acid, attack the teeth and promote decay.

FINAL RESUME

Longevity should be the rule and not the exception.

For the benefit of those who seek health and wish to profit through the application of natural laws, I would lay down the following rules which should be conscientiously observed:

The proper procedure for the uninformed, those who have no knowledge of themselves, is to first place themselves in the hands of competent *physicians and dentists.*

To determine the cause of your physical troubles, *begin at the beginning.*

Go to an alert, progressive dentist. Have a detailed examination and X-rays made of the teeth and jaws to determine just what the conditions of the mouth are and what treatment is necessary.

Have X-ray plates made of the entire head and ascertain as nearly as possible the conditions of the areas in and around the ethmoid and sphenoid bones, the antrum and the frontal sinuses.

After having these examinations made, consult an expert diagnostician, one who specializes exclusively in diagnostic work. Have a thorough and complete organic diagnosis, urine-analysis, blood test and an analysis of the fecal matter. Regardless of how strong you think your lungs are, have a fluoroscopic examination of them made. In spite of vigorous health and apparent immunity from lung diseases, adhesions are frequently found in the lungs. This is true even of athletes.

Even if you have found nothing alarming in the tests made thus far, do not neglect giving attention to the spine. I have never yet seen a case where the spine was so perfect that it did not need some treatment. Have X-rays made to determine whether there is any dislocation of vertebrae, thickening of bones, curvature, or impingement of nerves. No matter how thorough the treatment, we cannot build health if the spine is dried and warped, the nerves pinched and the vertebrae displaced. Aside from the acids, produced by foods, which are responsible for these conditions, there are also childhood injuries, falls, jars and shocks which may have seemed insignificant at the time but constitute the cause of serious trouble later in life.

After the completion of these various examinations, you should be well informed as to your exact physical condition. You now have the basic knowledge necessary for health. You have learned the disorders and diseased conditions with which you have to battle. The next step is to eliminate them.

Have your dentist completely repair your mouth, if it is necessary. Overlook no decayed or abscessed teeth, pyorrhea conditions or imperfectly fitting and articulating crowns, bridges and plates. Get the services of the most efficient dentist you can find. The best dentist is not always the most expensive one (although the conscientious, efficient dentist deserves to be well paid). Neither is the dentist with the widest reputation always the expert he is proclaimed.

If there are any conditions to be corrected in the head, nose and throat, consult specialists in those lines.

Have any and all diseased vital organs treated by the attending physician or surgeon. I do not advocate surgical procedure except in extreme cases where the degenerated conditions of one or more organs threaten the involvement of others and the life of the patient. Discriminate surgery is often the means of prolonging life for a number of years. Indiscriminate operations have abruptly terminated thousands of lives.

The foundations of health are now established, and the next step is to learn the way of Right Living which will build and maintain physical perfection. Eat the foods as they grow in their natural raw state, energized by the sun and air. Do not destroy their power and life-giving elements by cooking and seasoning them with condiments. Eat raw vegetables, fruits, nuts, and drink plenty of milk and cream.

Exercise daily in the fresh air.

Take brisk walks at least every day.

Sleep nine hours or more, every night, getting at the very least two hours before midnight.

Each day drink one glass of water to every fifteen pounds of your weight and all in addition to this amount which you may desire.

Keep the bowels regulated with laxative fruits and vegetables.

Resort to a pure mineral oil whenever necessary.

Never be guilty of excesses and you will achieve mental and physical equilibrium.

Practice moderation in all things.

To prevent recurrence of your former troubles after you have established Health:

1. Visit your dentist at least every four months. If there has been an extreme condition existent in your mouth, see the dentist every third month.

Gum diseases necessitate constant vigilance, and the examinations of the mouth must be regulated according to the severity of the case and the strength of the patient.

2. Have a complete organic examination once a year, with an analysis of the urine and a blood test.

3. Have an examination and X-ray of the spine made annually.

4. Make it a point to visit an expert osteopath, chiropractor, naprapath or masseur, whichever one is indicated, not less than twice a year. The manipulation of the spine and various joints will keep the body pliable, assist the circulation by preventing impingement of the nerves and circumvent any tendencies to spinal disorders.

I would advocate just as detailed attention to the child, to guarantee its growth and perfect development. Often the neglected injuries of childhood are more serious than the parent realizes and result in serious ailments later.

This may all seem a lengthy procedure to insure Health, but *disease prevention* is cheaper physiologically and financially than *disease contraction,* which costs both life and money.

2943277

Made in the USA